Essential Gut & Hormone Wellness

Finding Balance Naturally

Essential Gut & Hormone Wellness

Finding Balance Naturally

TERI A. RINGHAM

Table of Contents

Disclaimer

The content in this book is for educational and informational purposes only, and it is not intended as medical advice. I am not a medical professional and cannot diagnose, treat, or prescribe. The information contained herein should not be used to diagnose, treat, prescribe, or prevent any disease or health illness. The author and printer accept no responsibility for such use. Please consult with a qualified, licensed health care professional before acting on any information presented here. Any statements or claims about the possible health benefits conferred by any foods, supplements, essential oils, or lifestyle changes have not been evaluated by medical professionals or the Food & Drug Administration.

Introduction

Take an eighteen-year-old girl (our beloved daughter Karly) on twelve medications enduring a revolving door of emergency room visits and four failed surgeries. Imagine the concern and frustration when doctors and specialists (including Mayo Clinic) tell her "all has been done that can be done." Consider her then 52-year-old mother (myself) with gut issues, fibromyalgia, lupus, and severe adrenal and thyroid issues with recommendations from doctors for several medications. Take an eighty-seven-year-old man (a beloved friend) with newly diagnosed prostate cancer and diabetes with a recommendation of chemical injections to shut down his hormones as well as several medications he will be using for the rest of his life.

Fast-forward several years to today. Same girl. Same mother. Same elderly man. Zero synthetic prescription medications. Each one is now leading and rejoicing in a normal life.

What changed? Our mindset and our approach to wellness were transformed. The same principles for each of us—although greatly different in age and gender—were used in our approach to wellness. The same approach resides within *Essential Gut & Hormone Wellness – Finding Balance Naturally.*

My journey into natural health practices was forced upon me—much as it is upon many of us—when it began as a result of watching our daughter suffer greatly from hormone-related issues beginning with her very first menstrual period. At the age of twelve, her cramping was so severe she slept on the bathroom floor due to the constant need to vomit. There were times

1

the cramping was so relentless, she would faint right in front of us, during school, extracurricular activities or while out with friends.

As her mother, watching her suffer was heartbreaking. Like any good parents would do, we eventually took her to the doctor seeking help. One of the first lines of defense used at the doctor's office for hormone issues in a female is a prescribed treatment of birth control pills (BCPs). Knowing what I know now, I would have refused synthetic hormone BCPs as an option, but, at the time, we had no reason to question her doctor's recommended treatment. Over the next few years, we unfortunately saw no improvement. Instead, her condition worsened to the point it was no longer five days of every month but thirty out of thirty days of every month. This escalated to more appointments, pills, surgeries, and a multitude of emergency room visits. Over a period of fifteen years, we watched a beautiful girl become a walking pill receptacle and a shell of the young female we once knew. Every day handfuls of pills were being put in her body. She endured four surgeries that gave no relief. She was not improving but instead spiraling into anxiety, night terrors, and depression. The time for change came as we watched her in seizures in the emergency room from the Gardasil vaccine strongly encouraged by her gynecologist. At this point, I realized handing our child over to doctors who obviously didn't have an answer for this condition yet continued to recommend treatments and surgeries was not the solution. It was time to start learning natural health options.

We went through four phases during this awful time before coming to the conclusion we were going to have to change our approach from sick care to health care.

Phase I: Listen

We were good patients in this phase and did everything as directed. I researched the best doctors and specialists. I begged to get into appointments sooner when we were told nothing was available for weeks or months and Karly was doubled over in pain. I made sure she took her medication as directed. We allowed the surgeries, the pills, and even horrific (in retrospect) toxic injections of a drug designed to shut down the female system and restart it once the drug is stopped. Little did I know, Lupron is also prescribed as a cancer drug that was never approved for female hormone treatments. Guess who didn't do her research prior to allowing her child to take it? I simply followed the doctor's recommendation without question and without research. One quick Google search would have easily provided multiple links to information backed by research to have made me question—and refuse—this toxic drug. Fifty lashes for me!

Phase II: Cry

At this point, it was becoming apparent what was being prescribed wasn't working, but we had no idea what else to do. This frustration and futility made us hit our breaking point. The need to relieve the stress of watching your child spiral downward led to only one response—cry.

Phase III: Question

We saw no improvement. Doctors, at this point, told us all that could be done for her endometriosis had been done. They had no more answers other than to suggest continuing the meds, increasing their dose, or enduring another surgery. Finally, we started to question and not accept the standard medical treatments. This, of course, was not well received in the doctor's office. I get that. Doctors are busy; they have pressure to see X number of patients per day, and the last thing they need is a parent questioning their prescribed treatment. However, on our side of the coin, we were completely frustrated with seeing our child spiraling into a disjointed treatment of drugs and surgeries. As the years went by and doctors were unable to give us solutions, we found it easier for them to blame the patient than to admit they didn't have the answer.

Phase IV: Change

The night we watched Karly in seizures on the floor of the emergency room as a reaction to a vaccine highly recommended by her gynecologist will forever be ingrained in my memory. Our hearts were in our chests in fear of losing her. Nothing was helping. She was only getting worse. If something didn't change, she would be dead. I had no doubt about that at this point. The number of narcotics, the brain medication affecting her mental health, and the poor results of surgeries were going to kill her. Even though I didn't know anyone with her condition and situation who had found answers through natural medicine, it became evident we needed to work her off the pills, injections, and surgeries.

Thus, our change to a different mode of treatment began. Armed with whatever knowledge I could find on her condition while continuing to devour any natural health information available in relation to hormone conditions, we began to work with the body rather than against it. We changed our thought process from believing medicines heal to the actual reality that medicine cannot heal. We had to alter our mindset from giving in to the fear factor of what could happen if she didn't follow prescribed treatment to no longer accepting them due to the reality of what was *literally* happening for ten full years.

The road to better health isn't always smooth. But we go where we are led. As I read and researched, I felt directed to focus on certain words or information that made total sense for our situation. Thankfully, the information obtained through research and put into practice enabled us to see enough results to give us encouragement to continue on this road.

Karly is now on zero synthetic meds. We haven't visited an emergency room in over a year. She leads a normal, joyful, and vibrant life. After fifteen years of struggles, this is something we never, ever thought would happen.

On the flip side, we now had a new patient in our family—me. The stress on my body and mind during the years of watching Karly's struggles naturally took its toll on my own health. Stress and a poor diet led to too much weight loss, overworked adrenal glands with blood tests showing H-Pylori, lupus, fibromyalgia, and atrial fibrillation (AFib). Life was not good at this point. My health was becoming as big a mess as hers. Surgery eased the AFib symptoms but my research showed it would return if my health remained in poor condition. Eventually, the habits and practices I researched while learning how to help Karly turned out to be very handy as they were the same things I needed to incorporate for my own health, even though our situations were vastly different in symptoms. While I didn't know it when I first started learning, our root cause (as we shall discuss shortly) was very similar. The same as it is for most of us!

As I approach my sixtieth birthday, my past health issues are resolved. I'm back to a healthy weight, taking zero medications, and as far as I know, the lupus, fibromyalgia, and H-Pylori are gone. To be honest, I haven't retested. Testing for these types of ailments, for me, is a thing of the past. If I tested positively now, I wouldn't do anything different than maintaining good gut health, eating a healthy diet, exercising, and decreasing stress as much as possible. Although I don't have blood tests to prove it, I believe anyone who knows me personally would be hard-pressed to think I still suffer from any of these former health issues.

Although we never know what curves life throws at us, I now know whatever that curve might be, each and every one of us should always search for answers that work with the body. We should supply the body then allow the body to do the job it was designed to do naturally—come to balance and heal.

Why Me?

Why *should* you take your valuable time to read this information from me? That's a good question! Most women I visit with through my lectures, consultations in my health coach business, and online presentations tell me they greatly value the information I offer as a badly needed road map for converting from modern medicine to natural health. They use this information as a guide from the beginning to show them where to focus in natural health options for their body, possible standard medicine options, and naturopath or functional medicine doctors' protocols. Standard medicine, a godsend in an emergency, leans heavily on pharmaceuticals for ongoing symptoms while natural medicine practitioners emphasize supplements, cleanses, and natural health—often to an amount the average person is completely overwhelmed.

My niche is sharing researched information that can help the average person, with no medical background, reduce the learning curve on the various types of doctors and natural health treatments on the market. I have been a speaker for large and small groups hungry to take charge of their health. I am certified in Reiki and hold certification from the Institute of Nutritional Leadership training program. Pharmacists, RNs, chiropractors, physicians' assistants, and MDs have either consulted with me for their health, requested information from my research, or utilized my advice to prescribe for their patient (my wellness client). Yes, there are times I recommend seeing your doctor!

I have logged thousands of hours of reading and researching with emphasis on working with the body to heal naturally through gut and hormone support. I have helped those struggling to navigate through the differences and expectations from their MD, naturopath or functional medicine doctor, chiropractor, or acupuncturist. I also suggest questions to ask, research to do prior to health/medical appointments, as well as information on natural health that may replace the need for a doctor appointment.

For essential oils users, there is a supplement at the back of the book on using our oils for body systems' support. I have been an oils "user" for over seven years, and I educate others at workshops and conferences for both small and large groups regarding the incorporation of essential oils for gut and hormone support. Many essential oils users are well versed in using oils but aren't necessarily familiar with the importance of focusing on gut health and insulin in the quest for wellness. While we hope oils can resolve health issues, in truth, as we shall see, we must have good gut health, diet, stress reduction, and insulin support as well as toxin removal to reach that wellness and balance. My experience is utilized within oils groups for information on insulin, gut health, hormone balance tips, diet, and toxins to heal the body and bring it to balance for wellness while also having extensive experience and information on the many ways we can use essential oils for support once wellness is achieved. The main content of this book is to help you understand how the body works and the methods that can heal and support your gut, hormone, and whole body health. The supplement on essential oils is to discuss how oils can help support and maintain that balance once it is achieved as well as some oils suggestions to consider for support specifically in the gut and hormone areas.

A key part of any health success story is the person seeking guidance and taking advantage of information provided. Without commitment and strong desire, it can be tempting to stray from the healing path. My goal with each person I consult and for this book is to provide motivation so you can make—and stick—to your commitment to healing naturally as much as possible. The need for someone who has discovered natural methods outside of the medical establishment is strong. Many today do not want medicines, and they don't want difficult protocols. However, they want someone familiar with standard medical care as well so they have a guide to what's extreme in their health care. They want guidance in the simplest format possible so they can stick to it. A health protocol program is much like an exercise program: if you don't keep it simple *and* enjoy it, you won't stick with it.

This book will guide you as you make the decision to pursue natural health care when you decide what you are doing is not working. It will also aim to help you avoid the medicine merry-go-round we were once on. I feel honored you chose my book for its information; I hope it might help you venture forth or reinforce your commitment to natural health. If you don't finish this book with a passionate desire to commit to clean living and learning all you can about your body, then I've failed.

But this isn't about me. It's about you and your family. It's about what can be done to incorporate natural health to help you live life as intended—with joy, passion, and vitality. Please read, absorb, and put into practice any of the information you find helpful for you and your family. It is my honor and pleasure to walk this path with you.

Why This Book?

Some of the books I love on natural health contain a few of the same principles I'll discuss. However, many of these books go into extensive research and in-depth detail that may be more than a person without a medical background that is seeking information wants to decipher. Consider this book as a road map for the average person to get started in caring for the body naturally. I hope to present this potential health-changing information in a way that helped me learn—in a simple, logical manner, focusing on a few areas instead of complicated protocols.

In this book, I plan to connect the dots for the reader on key areas of supporting the human body so we can act accordingly to provide that support. When we focus on these key areas to begin our health-improvement journey, we sometimes bring other parts of the body into line without extensive testing, heavy cleanses, or intensive treatment. We allow the body to take back what was taken from it over the years—its natural ability to heal, to come to balance. We will discuss ways we might bring into balance to one area of the body especially a master part of the body to relieve the stress on other body parts that may have had to kick into high gear to compensate for the out-of-balance master hormone or gland further up the chain. As the master's stress is relieved, the poor, overworked fellas further down the line may be given a badly needed break. They are given the opportunity to ease back into good health on their own instead of forcing them with treatments or medicine. This simple concept—start with the master hormone and work your way down—has worked well for our family and many others with whom I consult. Working to balance (homeostasis) is something the body does naturally when provided with the proper tools. We will discuss these tools within *Essential Gut & Hormone Wellness.*

Is it simple? In a way...yes. It is surely easier when we focus on a few key areas rather than the complexity of micromanaging blood levels, hormone levels, and focusing on individual glands and organs further down the line from the root problem—often the gut or insulin levels. The intrinsic human body interactions are not simple, but we can make healing it less complicated by looking to root cause rather than trying to deal individually with the resulting array of symptoms the body sends us.

In this book, we will:

- Look at the cause of gut and body inflammation with some simple steps to ease this inflammation.
- Discuss blood sugar and insulin and ways to help bring balance.
- Learn the extreme influence diet has on our behavior and our overall health.
- Consider diet changes that make a big impact on healing our body and brain health.
- Study the impact lifestyle diet and toxins have on hormone and overall body systems' disruption plus easy ways to avoid or remove these toxins.
- Offer ways to ease stress and emotional responses to avoid the damaging effect emotions can have on overall health.

It's important each of us learns these areas to care for our family and ourselves. If we don't, here's what I've seen happen in the real world. People decide to really commit to their health and go one of two directions. They go the route of western medicine, which involves expensive and invasive testing along with a grocery list of medications. Or they go holistic and natural health and find a natural health-based professional who might also run an array of blood tests, tissue levels, H. pylori, Lyme testing, etc. The problem with prescribed medications is we don't usually get information on what might be the root cause of the health condition so we never know to stop the habit that may be causing it. Therefore, we often come back to get a different med or more meds. With the more holistic approach, we might get products for cleanses, numerous nutritional supplements, and vitamin programs without a clear understanding of why we are using them or how to use them resulting in information overload.

It can become very discouraging when we rely *more* on tests and supplements than focusing on diet, gut health, and support of healthy insulin levels. When we narrow our focus to gut health and insulin balance first this normally involves less information to absorb. This makes it more manageable for each of us to eventually expand our learning to why we are using certain foods, practices, and supplements to accomplish our purpose.

You may have to take a little extra time and effort to prepare your foods, to find products with fewer chemicals, and to avoid stressors that damage the body, but this is far more beneficial than following a pill regimen and/or invasive procedures. If you make an honest effort, you will see and feel at least some, if not great, improvement.

Why this book? Because what I hear and see repeatedly is the need for less complicated instruction and simple information. As I sat in the chair of my local salon earlier today, I heard the words, "I don't want all kinds of complicated protocols, programs, and information. I just want someone to tell me what to do!" This is the purpose of my book. While not intended to "tell", it is meant to guide and give you understanding and focus while you use it to lead you on the path to better health through caring for your body naturally.

Getting Started

Much of the information I will discuss comes from years of extensive research of online health articles from both medical and natural health websites as well as a multitude of natural health books and seminars. It also comes as a result of information I found helpful from my appointments with naturopaths, acupuncturists, and chiropractors. My goal is to hopefully cut a few years off your learning curve by offering you this information in a condensed and refined version that you likely will not be given at a doctor appointment while giving you details that may help support and retain what might have been discussed at your naturopath or functional medicine doctor appointment. If you find your eyes glazing over in boredom (heaven forbid!) or information overload during our discussions in this book, I recommend you return to the main focus points that will be listed in each section of the book.

Getting started means becoming very aware of the body's way of speaking to us through the symptoms—or messages—it sends us. Our symptoms are warning signs that our bodies are overloaded and need help. We tend to ignore the symptoms and continue to push our stressed body, or we go to the doctor hoping for some help. The help often comes in the form of medications that mask our body's messages to us—our symptoms. And we know what happens from there...

Do you function normally when you are sick with a cold or the flu? No, you very likely do not. We usually feel pretty awful and find it difficult to even get out of bed. The last thing we want are demands on us. And you can bet we aren't going to respond well to those demands if we get them. Now imagine your body's cells, organs, and glands being constantly sick due to our poor eating habits and toxic environment. The body parts become stressed and inflamed. Even though they send out symptoms to say they don't feel well, we continue to place demands (many times excessive demands) on them while at the same time continuing our damaging habits of consuming the standard American diet and using chemically laden personal care or home products. How can our body parts *possibly* function normally? Imagine this state of sick for your gut, brain, thyroid, joints, ovaries—all greatly affected by inflammation.

Over the years, the body compensates repeatedly and allows us to neglect proper diet, proper lifestyle, and while living in a chemically laden environment. However, at some point, it all culminates. Many times, this occurs at the time of a major life event such as childbirth, employment changes, perimenopause, house sale, menopause, divorce, or perhaps caring for a loved one with serious health issues. This places increased stress on an already stressed body, and we hit our breaking point.

The body tells us it is on overload through symptoms such as eczema, diarrhea, anxiety, depression, migraines, allergies, and more. If we get medicines to deal with the body's messages through these symptoms, we are telling the body to stop talking to us. This is a grave mistake. Yes, it will stop talking...for a while. Meanwhile, what's going on within the body once we block its message is critical. The root cause of the problem will be brewing and manifesting in other body parts or systems, and it *will* reemerge at some point with likely even worse issues. The human body—your body—will only speak through a smaller voice (a symptom) for so long before we get our wake-up call from the body in a louder voice (a serious health condition). Normally, this is the point where we place ourselves in the hands of the medical world to be fixed. We haul ourselves (or children) to the doctor for help. Ideally, that's exactly what we should do. However, our current health care system has been trained to distribute medicine to continue to shut down or block the gland or organ's message to us or, worse, cut it out. If that treatment fails, we are prescribed medicines to suppress our immune system. This doesn't just block messages, it will completely shut down our body's way of speaking.

We received the wake-up call for Karly. As her parent, I became determined to absorb any information I could find that made sense for her symptoms. As it turned out, the principles I was learning and applying for her were the same ones eventually needed to turn my health around. These basic principles helped both of us at greatly different ages. They were used by my eighty-seven-year-old male family friend with diabetes and prostate cancer. Young or old. Male or female. These methods have been used to help many others as the body works to balance (homeostasis) with good— sometimes great—results.

Does it happen overnight? Good gosh no. We don't get sick overnight, so we can't expect to get better quickly. However, if we do our due diligence toward repairing the gut and eating well, we might see some of the symptoms be alleviated fairly quickly (sometimes within days). Just because symptoms might ease, however, this does not mean the root cause was healed. It means we've started but haven't finished the job. Symptoms may subside, but we still must address *why* we have them or they will return... sometimes with a vengeance. Therefore, we ease the warning signs while working on the root causes we will discuss in this book.

Natural health relief, while proven and powerful, is still doubted by many. Do you doubt that simple, natural remedies can possibly be powerful enough to be the answer for your child or your situation? That's completely normal and understandable. I felt the same way at one time. Feeling this way led us to many years of pain and sorrow that delayed our taking control of our health. If you question the ability of natural care to help you or your child, I recommend to always remember the potential alternative if we don't give natural health a shot—the possibility of the revolving door of medical appointments, meds (and more meds), or even surgery. What would it hurt to come from the other direction and see if we can't find the root cause? Let's remove the powerful forces damaging the body and let it heal.

The goal must be to fully embrace changes that help us improve; this is a lifestyle, not a temporary treatment. Upon adopting this lifestyle, most of us feel so much better that we do *not* want to return to the old ways. However, if you're sliding, remind yourself of the ultimate outcome: a return to your old state of body health.

Embrace the changes we'll discuss. Make them your new and continued way of life. God gave you *one* body... only one. The human body has a big forgiveness curve. It really was not designed to be sick or out of balance any more than you want to be sick or out of balance. Offer it the care and respect it so richly deserves. Focus on the basics we will discuss and incorporate them. When you give your body what it needs for good health, your body will get to work on doing the job it knows best: to repair, regenerate, and ultimately reward *you* with good health. You'll know you're on the right track when you begin feeling less stress, more balance, and more energy. Most importantly, you will not only feel but you will *be* more empowered in your mind and body. And *that* is a fabulous place to be!

Chapter One: The New Normal

It's fairly common in today's health care system to be told our health condition is normal, inherited, part of being a female, or part of getting older. Therefore, we should simply accept our circumstances, take the prescribed meds, allow the suggested surgery, and learn to live with it. Before we decide to just live with our condition or accept it as normal, let's look at some quick statistics:

- IBS (irritable bowel syndrome) affects 15% of people in the United States (www.aboutibs.org).

- In the United States, 29 million people (9.3%) have diabetes, according to the Centers for Disease Control and Prevention.

- National Health and Nutrition Examination Survey claims from 2003 to 2012, the percentage of adults 40 and over using a cholesterol-lowering medication increased from 20-28%.

- Approximately 39.6% of men and women will be diagnosed with cancer of any site at some point during their lifetime based on 2010-2012 data from the National Cancer Institute entitled "Seer Stat Fact Sheet."

- The CDC states 1 in 4 women of reproductive age is on a depression medication.

- Endometriosis affects 176 million women worldwide and 1 in 10 females (10%) in the United States between the ages of 12-54 (www.nuff.org).

- It is estimated that polycystic ovarian syndrome (PCOS) affects about 8-10% of women of reproductive age, according to www.womenshealth.gov.

- 10.9% of women ages 15-44 have fertility issues, according to www.womenshealth.gov.

- By the age of sixty, one-third of women have a hysterectomy (www.nuff.org).

Take a good hard look at these numbers. Now look at your family and decide which person and which one of these statistics will apply to them. If you have at least three people in your family, you will be impacted by at least one of these statistics. If you have four members, the number increases. Five members and it's almost a guarantee to have at least one member with a serious health condition. Which disease or condition will end up applying to our loved ones? Do we have to sit back and accept it happening to one of our family members? Do these statistics seem *normal*? Did we see them in our grandparents or great-grandparents' day? You can bet we most surely did not. Why isn't our government, our health care system, or *someone* more outraged over these startling statistics? They should be. *We* should be. Even if you are blessed to avoid being a statistic, the odds are extremely high someone you love is or will be affected with one of these conditions. Sadly, these statistics are getting worse despite the miracle of modern medicine. Although health care in the United States is the most expensive in the world, (based on patients' and physicians' survey results on care experiences and ratings on various dimensions of care), we ranked last of eleven major countries, according to The Commonwealth Fund's 2014 article "Mirror, Mirror on the Wall: How the Performance of the U.S. Healthcare System

Compares Internationally, 2014 Update." The April 2010 edition of *International Journal of Obesity* claims, our children's generation is the first generation predicted to have a shorter lifespan than their parents.

We hear of the miracle of modern medicine and, in an emergency, it can be a miracle. But for day-to-day life and the billions of dollars poured into our medical schools, clinics, high-tech equipment, specialists, and lab facilities... where's the miracle? Why don't we see declining disease statistics, and *why* do so many of us struggle with day-to-day health?

It's Not Working

Sometimes the most difficult part of making the transition to alternative/natural health is to accept that it can actually work. At first, when I read articles or had friends share information regarding natural options for helping with major health issues, I never considered this information as a replacement for medicines and doctors' advice. We tend to think medicine is powerful and necessary while lifestyle changes must be too simple to be effective. After all, if basic changes work why don't we know about it? Why doesn't our doctor tell us?

To be honest, in most cases, your doctor truly does not know; it is not a part of medical school education and it's much more face-saving to negate alternative natural care rather than saying "I don't know". Under our current health system, to ask your doctor about supplements or methods of natural care is asking for a response that many times minimizes natural health methods. At best, your doctor tells you go ahead saying, "It likely won't help but can't hurt."

The common mode of thought in "modern" medicine for health issues is when all else fails (and it will if we don't look at the root cause), blame genetics. It's in our genetics so there's nothing we can do about it. This mindset tends to be "my grandparents and parents had diabetes so therefore, I must have diabetes" or whatever the health condition might be. Thus, if we eventually have diabetes, we accept it as our destiny, continue our diet overloaded with sugars and grains and take our medicine as prescribed to continue down the road of premature illness and death rather than changing our lifestyle.

For many conditions, we do not have to accept this. Genetics are powerful indeed, but we have the ability to exert influence on our genetics in not only a bad—but also good—direction. Epigenetics is our influence on the body's cells through our diet, our toxins, our stress, and our chemical levels to improve upon the genetic predisposition. If genetics were the key component causing the skyrocketing statistics of today's prominent health conditions, why didn't our grandparents have a higher statistic as well? Yes, we can be prone to certain diseases or conditions, but our influence to enact that disease or condition within the cells has been greatly minimized in our society, health systems teachings, and thought processes. There is not nearly enough discussion on the dramatic change in our environment and diet since our grandparents' day. We cannot put complete blame on our genetics while, at the same time, ingesting unprecedented amounts of sugars and grains. To accept and blame genetics for our health condition means we take the "it's not with my control" path and also consent to taking meds for the rest of our life. And that should be a very sobering thought.

The big issue is how and why we have strayed so far in our current and trusted health system. Why does it continue to prescribe, cut, and inject while current statistics continue to escalate showing this is clearly not working? Even worse, why do we, as patients, continue to subject ourselves to this type of treatment? At most doctor appointments, we are asked why we are there and given a label for some type of medical condition or disease for our symptom; your doctor rolls his or her chair over to the computer, brings up the list of meds for that issue, and away you go in eight minutes or less with a prescription that has two pages of listed side effects. Is this medical care? Or is this sick care? Were you asked about your lifestyle, toxin exposure, diet, activity level, or emotional state? Very likely you were not. Thus, it's also very likely you will be back to that doctor's office because the meds you were just prescribed will create a new condition in you. This works well for the profit line but not so well for you or me *or* our loved ones.

Why can't our doctors discuss gut lining damage, toxin interference with our body organs, or insulin levels to work toward hormone balance? Honestly, because this type of information is not taught to them. This is not all the doctor's fault. Many go into this field with wonderful intentions of healing people. On the way through medical school, they are given a tremendous amount of information on the human body interactions to learn and absorb. This is all good and, of course, we count on them learning about the human body at a much deeper level than we could ever learn. That's what doctors do, right? They learn about the body and then instruct us on what we should do to get better when we have a health condition.

Here's where the problems first begin. In today's medical schools, a huge proportion of students' time is spent in class repeatedly given instruction on the "miracle" of medicines to help the body's interactions. Unfortunately, while doctors attend lectures and study in medical school on this miraculous science of mankind (aka pharma) creating medicines to help the body, they fail to receive lectures on nutrition, toxin avoidance, and

21

stress reduction. A study conducted by the department of nutrition at the University of North Carolina at Chapel Hill published in 2010 shows that only about one-quarter of more than one hundred medical schools surveyed provided the twenty-five hours of nutrition instruction recommended by the National Academy of Sciences in 1985—more than twenty-five years ago. Twenty-five hours of nutrition in 8-10 years of schooling with only one quarter of the schools even meeting this lowly requirement? This makes it pretty obvious why we aren't getting diet and natural health information at our medical appointment.

The information taught in medical school includes all the anatomy and science on the human body as well as extensive lectures, presentations, and information on how and why prescription drugs work. But much of this information is influenced by a medical school receiving millions of dollars in contributions from pharmaceutical companies. Thus, these students-our eventual doctors sincerely believe this is the way to deal with human conditions and illnesses. When our health professionals are trained to believe this, they influence us to also have this same mindset. The white coat syndrome of respecting and accepting all decisions on our health care is a powerful influence that ends with having our treatment (usually involving prescriptions) dictated to us rather than discussing options to prevent the condition.

Another aspect to consider is that our medical system is insurance driven—both for insurance to pay for your doctor visits and insurance for the doctors to cover themselves if they are sued. This has a major effect on how we are treated. Our medical insurance covers our doctor bills. They don't pay for things such as classes on digestive health or a thermography (versus mammography) appointment. Therefore, because we want our appointments paid, we are literally directed toward the treatment decided from an insurance industry that covers pharmaceuticals but not health care education.

In addition, malpractice insurance is directing what our doctor can and cannot do. If your doctor told you to eat healthy food to help bring down your blood pressure instead of prescribing a blood pressure medication but you continued poor eating habits and had a stroke, the doctor has been set up for a potential lawsuit. The standard protocol for high blood pressure is a blood pressure medication. Since he did *not* prescribe it to you as the protocol recommended, there's a potential lawsuit for that doctor. His insurance rates may greatly increase since he did not follow protocol thus becoming a higher risk from an insurance industry's point of view. So when you ask your doctor about holding off on a medication while you work to improve your test results, the doctor is in a conundrum.

It has been ingrained in us since childhood watching our parents follow this system. Thus, it's the system we know and follow as well. Therefore, it's difficult to get people to change direction and accept that some things, while possibly good for them, are going to cost money out of pocket. Unless we can get past the mindset that health care for our bodies must be paid for by insurance, we cannot escape the current health care system.

Please know I am not here to discourage medical care and doctors when they are needed. There are many caring professionals in the health care field who truly do want to help. In an emergency, our doctors and nurses and medicines can be lifesavers, and that is the time we can see the miracle of modern medicine. For body *conditions* rather than emergencies, however, there is a vast difference in treatment between natural health care and medical health professionals. Our health care system is working *against* the body rather than *with* the body.

Due to this mindset and lack of belief in working naturally with the body, nearly 70 percent of Americans are taking one or more prescription drugs for a chronic medical condition and more than half receive at least two prescriptions according to a 2013 article, "Age and Sex Patterns of Drug Prescribing in a Defined American Population" (www.mayoclinicproceedings.org). For a good number of these users, this means medication on a daily basis for, very likely, the rest of their lives.

Nature vs. Synthetic

Just because using a medication or drug has become normal in our society, let's not devalue the word medication or drug. A medicine *is* a drug. It will work in the body in a way to alter, block, or shut off the undesired symptoms. Because the human body works intrinsically, we can *never* alter or treat one part of the body without altering others' body systems. Thus, when we use a drug, we are altering not just the symptom but the entire body. This is one reason for the extensive list of potential side effects with each medication. If we study the human body, we understand there is no way we will ever instruct it to heal or correct itself by using medications on a long-term basis. The fact that 70 percent of our population relies on them is a reflection of the insidious infiltration into our medical schools thus into our health care field by pharmaceutical companies.

While we think medicine is more powerful, around 70 percent of all new drugs introduced in the United States in the past twenty-five years have been derived from natural products, reports a study published in the March 23 issue of the *Journal of Natural Products*. Therefore, drug companies often look to nature to create their medicine. A prescription medicine must have a synthetic component or it cannot be patented and sold by the pharmaceutical company manufacturing it. We cannot patent something natural such as a plant or herb. These drugs often come from a plant (nature's medicine) only to be altered synthetically so they can be patented and to force absorption into the cells. In our mindset and the marketing of medication, creations from a laboratory are supposedly more effective and better for us than nature's medicine. We tend to forget that *anything* created in a laboratory is a synthetic. A synthetic *is* a foreign substance to the body; something not accepted willingly by our cell receptors. Therefore, for our body to absorb and accept it, the substance needs to have components that help force it into the cells or interfere with a process in a way that is unnatural to the body systems. Each time we force the body, we may block a symptom but we also create an undesirable chain of reactions within the brain and body. Once again, this is part of the reason for the lengthy list of potential side effects enclosed on the package of any medicine we pick up at the pharmacy.

The body recognizes a natural component such as a plant or plant nutrient. It recognizes the nutrients, constituents, and enzymes in our food to readily accept and utilize it for the body interactions. I liken foods, vitamins, and nutrients as a tap on the cell door. If the cell needs that constituent, the door is opened to readily accept it. If not, as a natural substance, the body can easily synthesize and break it down to excrete that constituent. Drugs may tap on the cell door, but the cell may not recognize the blend of chemical constituents and refuse to absorb it. Therefore, the lab must create a blend of chemicals and constituents to help force the substance into the cell receptor—a rap on the door, so to speak. A tap on the door versus a rap on the door. If you are the cell, which would you prefer? Which do you think would be less disruptive to a cell that *will* have a reaction—good or bad, depending on the way its delivered to set off a series of reactions throughout the body? Again, the reason we have a long list of potential side effects. Forced versus welcomed, tap versus rap. There's a big difference.

A Different Approach

Most of us (including myself) do not have a medical degree or background that is the standard as the higher power in knowing how to help our bodies. And that's OK. Sometimes I wonder if we aren't a tad better off without that scientific background. This allows us to view the body as an intrinsic whole, the way it *should* be approached, instead of focusing on the scientific side of things. Currently, we go to this or that specialist for one part in our body giving us issues with little regard to our mental state, diet, or our environment even though each of these is a vital component in human health. Our condition rarely originates in a microcosm but rather originates much further "up the line" in the body from where it manifests. And unless we address the issue causing the symptom, we are likely putting a Band-Aid on the one area being treated.

An example of whole body interactions might be thyroid issues that cause symptoms such as weight gain, thinning hair, skin problems, or low energy. If we go to the doctor, he will test our thyroid, tell us the hormone secretion levels are out of range, and prescribe a medication. This is something the medication will (ideally) control but cannot cure; that's not within the medicine's abilities. Its function is to attempt to *control* the symptom or replace a natural body constituent. Therefore, it's extremely likely you *will* be on a med for your thyroid for the rest of your life. (Remember, this med has its long list of side effects). For many women, if the medicine is used but the thyroid worsens or perhaps has nodules, lasering it or cutting it out of our body becomes a possible treatment. If the thyroid is partially or totally removed, we need a medication to control the functions of the body that the thyroid used to do, right? If we go to the doctor for thyroid symptoms, it's highly likely we are now stuck on a lifetime of meds—a medicine that a lab created intending to replace the naturally intelligent, intrinsic interactions of the thyroid gland with our body systems.

Did we stop to consider *why* that thyroid has nodules or its hormone production is not at the correct levels? What if the gut lining is damaged, allowing toxins into the bloodstream and inflaming our organs-including our high susceptible Thyroid gland as well as many other glands to cause a myriad of symptoms and issues? What if the body is being exposed to chemicals and toxins affecting the thyroid? Did that medication or surgery solve these issues? No, it did not. Therefore, we *will* be back eventually (sometimes very quickly) to the doctor with a different symptom, a new problem—one created by the medication or lack of removal of the inflammation. Unless we resolve the inflammation affecting the body, a med, a surgery, or an injection, just won't do it. They cannot and will not solve the root cause of the imbalance. Thus, the imbalance will continue to manifest in our most susceptible body part.

Every body imbalance, condition, pain, or malfunction originates somewhere. For most of us, we can look to the condition of our gut, diet, stress levels, and environmental toxins to find these are major contributors to our imbalances, symptoms, and conditions. At the very least, it should be the first place to look before blocking or attempting to control a symptom. Even someone with a severe, inherited health condition can find some benefit from focusing on these areas. If we focus on finding and helping the imbalance, we should see some, if not great, improvement. You do not have to have a medical degree to know what the body needs at a cellular level. This more likely requires some basic knowledge and, truthfully, a whole lot of common sense. Every time you eat or drink, you are either feeding a negative cell reaction or a positive reaction. We offer toxins or disruptors through meds, soda, chips, processed foods, *or* we offer healing components in greens, fruits, healthy fats. "You are what you eat" is not just a catchy phrase. You *are* what you eat. This applies to you, your children, your parents, and to each and every one of us. Rocket science this most definitely is not. Keep the visual every time you lift your hand to your mouth. Is what's going in positive or negative to the body and thus, your body functions? Consider the last time you actually ate a vegetable (packaged mini carrots or iceberg lettuce don't count). Now consider if you are getting even one vegetable per day. It's a sad fact of the American diet that most of us are far away from getting our recommended amount per day.

As a little eye-opener for yourself, start being conscious of your (or your child's) intake of vegetables for a few days. Ask yourself, "Did I (my child) eat even one vegetable today?" We can't be perfect in our eating habits all the time, but let's be honest... there's a whole lot of truly awful going on in most of our eating habits. If we want health change, we need to improve what we eat. Even if you are a fairly healthy eater but have some type of health struggle, there's obviously still room for improvement.

The human body really does have an amazing gift of reaching

homeostasis with the proper diet and environment. It works every second of every day to balance, to heal, to function, and to create the perfection of the human body. Do we tell the body to heal a cut on our leg? Do we tell it to send the nutrients, enzymes, and minerals necessary to mend a broken bone? No, we don't. It simply needs proper nutrients through our diets. It needs us to stop the intervention and disruption of body systems by removing and avoiding the chemicals with which it is bombarded daily. It needs the stress relief of yoga, meditation, quiet time, exercise, and prayer to avoid the damage continued on not only the emotions but also the physical parts of the body such as our digestive and endocrine/hormone systems.

Was any of this discussed in your medical appointment? Sadly, there's an extremely high chance it wasn't. We've been conditioned to accept the unacceptable. We've been conditioned to accept a synthetic is better for fixing our bodies than God-given, pesticide-free food and a clean environment. We've been conditioned to rely on experts who have been trained in sick care rather than health care. And that's just unacceptable. You are *not* broken. You are *not* a pill receptacle. You are very likely *not* genetically inclined to live with an illness the rest of your life. However, you are likely in need of care. True care. Genuine care. Health care where you are asked *why* you have this symptom rather than prescribed a pill.

Believe

The professionals in our health care system most surely are not lacking intelligence. There are brilliant minds in the medical field. But brilliance does not always equate to intelligence or common sense. What our medical system *is* lacking is a huge component in the field of healing—the belief in the human body's abilities to balance. Through their schooling and the drug-

and insurance-driven system within which they must conform, they never learned—or have lost—hat belief.

No, the medical industry is most surely not slow of mind. But the truth is they have become greatly influenced to become slow of heart. And being slow of heart has led to interference with their ability to:

- Believe the human body needs less synthetic intervention and more support.

- Believe in the power of exercise to increase circulation and thus, increase healing.

- Believe when we offer the body nutrients while removing disruptors and toxins, the human body takes over to work toward homeostasis.

- Believe in the power of prayer, meditation, and stress relief.

- Believe when God created the human body, He created an amazing being with the innate, miraculous ability to balance and function in good health.

Since our medical system has either never learned or has lost the ability to believe, it falls upon each of us to believe. The beliefs listed above that we would love our doctors to have are the same beliefs each of us needs to acquire if we are going to help ourselves heal. You have the right to choose to believe in the body's innate ability to repair, or you can choose to believe the fear factor so many of us are subjected to at the doctor's office. As you work up the courage to tell your doctor you are going to hold off on using the medicine he/she just prescribed for you or your child for a chronic condition, one of the first responses is a myriad of potential, awful things that can happen if you don't take the prescribed treatment. It's worked on me, and it's worked on millions. Doctors aren't doing this to be evil. They truly believe it. Going down *that* road of fear and doing everything recommended only to spiral down in health is not at all pleasant. I've watched it happen in my daughter and in my own health. I've watched it in good friends and total strangers. One illness *will* lead to another if we don't get to the root cause. If a surgery, injection, or medication will truly *heal* or take care of the situation, then by all means do it. But also know this... We thought, we hoped, we prayed every specialist, every medicine, every injection or surgery would help our extremely sick child as well. But it didn't. And you know why? Because we were not getting to the root cause. We did not know at the time, but we do now, that her gut health was awful, her diet was awful, her toxin exposure (thus, her xenoestrogens) were through the roof, and her insulin was completely out of control causing her emotions, hormones, and pain levels to be severely affected. What surgery or pill could possible help this? The inflammation in the body was so great and so advanced, how could we ever think medical intervention would solve the problem?

And therein is the fallacy of modern medicine today and the influence it has on our common sense. Until the moment we were faced with little alternative, it finally became clear that ultimately *we* (and especially she) had to make lifestyle changes to get the damage and inflammation under control. She had to make the changes that involved a focus on diet, healing gut lining, and hormone balance. This is the difficult part for so many. We want to turn it over to someone to fix us because medicine is not our area of expertise. Plus it's darned hard to change our daily habits that we like. It's only natural to want to put our health in the hands of the professionals. We should be able to do this. But in this day with this system we have labeled health care, we can't. The hope is, as we have more doctors disillusioned with the current system, we will see more venturing into the natural and alternative care fields such as naturopaths and functional medicine doctors. If you have or find health professionals on board with this type of care being their main focus, hold onto them as your health advisors. However, whether its traditional or natural medicine, we must always remain as the driver—the one in control of the decisions in our health care. They advise—we decide.

I have had people deny the possibility to heal (or greatly improve) their health naturally saying, "I'm (my child) is sicker than the average sick person" or "I have too much wrong with me to heal." I understand being frustrated and without hope. I understand the thought process of being too sick for natural health. We were once at the same point. We had to see our daughter in seizures to accept that perhaps there was a better way than twelve prescription medications on an eighteen-year-old girl.

What if we had not eventually believed in the power the human body holds? Where would we be today? The same can apply for you and your family. Do not assume or lose hope because you think your condition is too unusual or you are sicker than those who have chosen to follow the natural medicine path. Please don't dismiss natural or alternative health help. None of us is too sick, too damaged, or too far gone. Because the human body will never cease to surprise us on what it can do to rebound and balance. For health concerns, it becomes very important that you own it, or it will own you. By owning it, you don't accept a label, you refuse to accept nothing more can be done, and you don't assume it's genetic so you will be living with it for life. You *choose* to become empowered through your own research and to take charge of your health rather than relying on someone you assume has more expertise than you.

With today's lifestyles and flawed medical system, for most health conditions, you first and foremost need to turn to the one true professional of your health... you. *You* work toward good diet and toxin removal. You learn what your body does and does not like. You pay attention to the body's symptoms. Nobody can learn and watch for you what your body needs and what your body's reactions are as well as you.

Should you consider what an expert tells you? Absolutely. Should you research to ensure it makes sense and you agree? Absolutely! But never lose sight of the important mindset that knowledge is power—the power to be the one determining the direction of your health. The fact you took the time to purchase and read this book shows you have resolved to be a decision maker in your health care. It also shows you care enough about yours and your family's health to take the time to learn all you can. Mega kudos to you!

I am thankful every single day that we were led to believe. Your purchase and reading of this book shows you are ready to believe as well. Whether your goal is to improve your foundation of good health habits or whether it's to help a loved one, start by absorbing every bit of information available regarding your particular health concern, wherever you can find it. Use it to enable you to continue on the path of good health, or if you are struggling, get *started* on the path to better health.

Getting stronger, working on getting well, living a truly vital and healthy life is a great future. Make the affirmations mentally. Make the root cause changes offered in this book. Then watch and *feel* the difference. Only when *you* believe—when *you* empower yourself to make positive lifestyle changes—can the power of the body to balance and heal itself begin.

The power is within *you*. It truly is. Research, learn, believe, and begin your journey!

Part One: Gut Health

Chapter Two: Eat Well to Be Well

The *ALL* mighty gut... It is mighty. And it is powerful in its influence on all other body systems in determining the state of our health. It's often difficult to comprehend just how much influence the gut has on overall health because we can't see or feel the interior body workings. Most of us will be hard-pressed to believe our digestive system has anything to do with our other health issues.

Focusing on digestive health to help ease whole body inflammation caused from toxins in our environment as well as foods causing gut lining damage can have a tremendous influence on pain, mental health, *and* hormone issues. When we have depression, anxiety, joint swelling, and hormone imbalance, it may not seem related to gut health. Yet, gut health is exactly where we need to look first.

I am still amazed and extremely grateful when I think back to where we *were* with Karly's health versus where we are today. The digestive system's influence on her health was a major source of her cramping and imbalances. These natural methods that I first considered ineffective turned out to be very powerful—even more than the twelve medications. Drugs are powerful but so is working on gut health. The difference is gut health repair can be healing.

One reason I believe we aren't resolving many of the health issues in America is because the majority of people are completely clueless just like we were. Because they do not suffer from acid reflux, nausea, diarrhea, constipation, or some other obvious symptom, most believe they don't have a compromised digestive system. This, unfortunately, is a common but sad mistake.

Gut Check

The digestive system encompasses the square footage of approximately one full tennis court. When that much area of the body gets inflamed and disrupted, it absolutely has to have an impact on whole body health. It is also one of twelve body systems. The body is a complicated, intrinsic machine with a symbiotic relationship of interactions and communications going on between all body systems at *all* times. Have no doubt, when we interfere with one system, we most certainly will alter all the others. One system may be more affected than others, but all are ultimately disrupted. The inflamed digestive system may show up as obvious digestive symptoms such as nausea, vomiting, diarrhea, and acid reflux. However, it may not be entirely obvious it's a gut issue in the resulting health issues such as aching knees or joints, anxiety, skin rashes, fatigue, allergies, brain fog, or hormone imbalances. These might all be health issues we blame on genetics without considering (or knowing) a gut condition could be involved.

Here's an example of the average person in everyday life. Jenny is a good friend who has struggled with bronchial infection issues for years. In addition, she is very prone to allergic reactions. Following the typical health care methods, her doctors have prescribed antibiotics and steroids continually for the six months. While she was on these meds, I would mention the destruction drugs can have on our gut health and how immunity (think bronchial infections in this case) is linked to our bacteria balance. We also discussed probiotics and their benefits, especially after antibiotic use. Unfortunately, Jenny would list all the reasons why it was necessary to take her medications, playing to the common fear factor of ceasing the regimen her doctor had prescribed. Since it's not my place to push my beliefs, I dropped the subject.

Recently, we went to a restaurant together. She ate the bread in a basket along with some cheese and pasta. It wasn't four bites into the meal that her eyes and tongue started to swell. We hightailed it out of the restaurant and raced to her home so she could use a popular allergy medicine. On the way, she told me she was tired of all these allergic reactions and made an appointment with an allergy specialist. Knowing we have been through the revolving door of specialists with our daughter in hopes of getting an answer and *not* getting an answer, I brought up the potential irritation that the bread or cheese might have caused in her digestive system to instigate her reaction. She replied that she always eats bread and cheese with her meals, and they don't bother her. (Note: she's been sick with bronchial infections as well as allergic reactions off and on for over a year while eating the bread [gluten] and cheeses [yeast and additives]). Yet, she was convinced these foods weren't allergens because she always eats them. Therefore, she turned to a specialist she believes will get to the bottom of her condition.

See the problem here? Jenny is either unaware of foods' connection and irritation to the gut, or she does not believe they could possibly cause her reactions. The specialist will likely do all kinds of expensive testing to give her a list of all the foods that give her allergic reactions. While it's good to know what irritating foods she should avoid, this doesn't answer *why* she's allergic to so many foods. So she will continue to react and have inflammation and bacteria imbalance with more infections and more medications. Her list of foods she is allergic to will likely grow each year.

37

This is the same scenario that's going on with our children, our parents, and ourselves in far too many cases.

So how can Jenny begin the healing process for her gut imbalance? If she has been on antibiotics for over six months, it's likely they have pretty much destroyed the microbiome and bacteria balance of the gut. With bacteria balance a vital component in our immunity, it would be highly beneficial for her to take pretty hefty amounts of probiotics (a microbiome and bacteria support supplement) as well as fermented foods such as kefir, sauerkraut, or yogurt to rebuild gut balance. One probiotic capsule per day just cannot do it. Without substantial support, her gut bacteria will never rebuild and rebalance on its own. She needs to be diligent in her use of probiotics as well as patient for recovery.

Jenny must also avoid foods that irritate her gut so her damaged gut lining can avoid inflammation and begin its healing process. Her food list from the allergist can be handy but if bread, sugar, and dairy aren't on the list, she should also remove them. If Jenny doesn't do these things, here's her likely scenario: As she eats the food that bothers her digestive system, the digestive lining gets irritated. Pretty soon, this large amount of space in the human body causes a reaction within the entire body. The reactions in the body are going to signal it's upset in whatever way it can. For some, it's swollen eyes. For others, it's aching joints or rushed trips to the bathroom. For someone else, it's sneezing or eczema and psoriasis, arthritis, MS, depression, or anxiety.

Sadly, I'm almost positive the specialist will not have the answers for Jenny. Unless she introduces a hefty amount of good bacteria in the form of probiotics and fermented foods to rebuild gut bacterial balance and avoid commonly known foods that damage the gut lining, I'm afraid the issues will not only continue, but they may likely escalate.

A Simple Change

This is the same scenario being repeated in one form or another all over America today. Way too often, we are starting at the end of the chain—medicines to deal with the infections and swelling from the reactions—rather than looking at the beginning of the chain and asking *why* her body can't handle certain foods while another person's can. In fairness to my friend, I understand why she doesn't consider focusing on gut healing. We had been in pretty much the same place. It took over a decade to decide what we were doing was definitely not working, just like Jenny's current issues with allergies and reactions.

Once we made that decision, we educated ourselves with information from research. What kept showing up in all my research was surprising but simple: gut health. Even though her issues at this point were anxiety, depression, and incredibly severe menstrual cramping, the information I found pointed to digestive lining repair, diet, toxin, and stress removal.

At some point, it all made sense. No hormones could balance, no cysts could stop swelling, and the excruciating pain would never stop as long as her digestive lining was inflamed. When we looked at her diet, she was consuming pretty much everything on the list of foods that inflame the gut, which ultimately inflamed the cysts. Thus, we started removing these disrupting foods and environmental toxins that caused inflammation with some unexpected, but welcome, changes.

So, when I sit and listen to Jenny and see her body reactions, I understand since we've been there. I also understand why, at this point in her life, she is not willing to consider or accept simple things can make big differences.

Our situation in our family, my friend's problem with her food reactions, and almost every single person I visit with on health issues, all have one thing in common: the need to take a hard look at diet, the need to take care of a major body system (the digestive system), and the need to avoid the toxins with which we are bombarded on a daily basis.

Back to Basics

Starting with digestive health should be great news. This way you can choose *one* area to improve and channel your energies. When you can work on one area, you become the specialist of your gut health. By doing this, here are some results you might see:

- *You* will have hope for health improvement and support.

- *You* will know *why* you or your child has these issues. (Knowing is key to committing to change!)

- *You* will know how to avoid damaging the gut.

- *You* will know how to help the gut and thus, help the body.

- *You* will know as much or more on healing the body through attention to digestive health than most modern medicine practitioners since the majority of them do not even agree that a damaged gut lining is the issue in many of today's health conditions.

- *You* will know potential causes of damage and where to start for gut health as well as why.

When *you* know, you become empowered to take charge of your health. When you become knowledgeable, you no longer have to rely on appointment desks to get you into the next, great specialist who will likely have no more answers for you than the last one.

Chapter Three: Gut Health

Over two thousand years ago, Hippocrates emphasized the importance of gut health and how greatly our gut health reflects our whole body health. Just because Hippocrates, considered the father of Western medicine, did not have a fancy laboratory and a slew of pharmaceutical agents at his disposal, does not mean his knowledge is outdated. It turns out, he was extremely intelligent, and his teachings apply every bit as much today as they did thousands of years ago. Hippocrates was, and through his writings still is, the master educator on the human body. The original Hippocratic oath recited by all physicians when they obtain their medical license *had* a portion that read, "With regard to healing the sick, I will devise and order for them the best diet, according to my judgment and means; and I will take care that they suffer no hurt or damage."

Ancient practitioners knew all those years ago what to do for our health. Devise and order the best diet. Unfortunately, it's been forgotten in our modern lifestyles and medical system. Parents used to raise their children providing nutrient-rich foods. Doctors and parents led by example and instruction on what food to eat and use for healing a sick body and maintaining a healthy, vigorous body. We no longer obtain this information at a doctor's office and, sad to say, not even at home. Many children watch and learn how to order fries at the drive-through and which aisle the Fruit Roll-Ups are located at the grocery store; yet aren't educated on the nutrition of their food. We have a duty to our children and ourselves to get back to the basics of not only gut health but caring for the body as God intended.

Digestive Functions

How and why do we consider gut health so important? We'll get into more detail as this chapter unfolds, but in a nutshell, our digestive system is the very foundation of our mental *and* physical health with many responsibilities every single day. Here are few of the functions it performs on a daily basis as part of the foundation of good health.

Digestion

Note the keyword within the word digestion is digest. If we don't digest our food properly, we are wasting a big benefit from our food. Food should be broken down to extract nutrients and eliminate the unnecessary parts (toxins). Have you ever really thought about how miraculous it is that we eat and somehow what we need is extracted and the things we don't need are sent out the chute? Nutrition. Without it, we die. Without it, we cannot and do not function well. Low energy, fatigue, exhaustion, illness. Maybe it's just a lack of nutrients. Perhaps breaking down food to absorb nutrients is every bit as important as adding in high-quality vitamins and minerals.

Immune System

The communication and interrelation between gut bacteria is beyond amazing. If we wanted to name a superstar of the human body that helped protect and defend us from bacteria and viruses, our microbiome would get the crown. Battling with illness and disease to support your immunity by up to 80 percent, our gut microbiome is an oft ignored defender that can provide us with good health when we give it the support it needs. We'll talk about a little pill—it's actually a capsule—you can use for this support plus the foods you should be eating for this hugely important gut function in our upcoming section on whole body bacteria/microbiome balance.

Inflammation

This topic alone can make me look like a hyped-up science nerd. When you get to the nuts and bolts of the digestive system lining *and* its potential to add or subtract inflammation in the body, it's downright exciting. Wouldn't it be impressive if you could help many of your body health conditions or problems by supporting gut health? Get ready to be impressed with your gut...because you can!

Toxin Filter

Our digestive system sorts and removes toxins from the body. What are toxins comprised of? Bacteria and microbiome that your digestive system, in its infinite wisdom and design, removes from your food and your body. If the toilet in your home backs up, you know how awful that smell can be. Now imagine if your body's "toilet" backed up or malfunctioned. Imagine if those things that were supposed to leave the body were in your bloodstream being absorbed by tissues, glands, and organs that were never designed to deal with these toxins. (That's the digestive systems job.) Would that have an impact on your health? Your gut *should* keep those nasty little fellas where they belong and move them out the chute into the toilet. However, if we have a compromised gut lining or leaky gut, some of these awful smelling (and toxic) invaders can permeate into our bloodstream to potentially reach every other part of your body (glands, organs, muscles, joints, even the brain). This causes the affected body part to become inflamed which leads to malfunction, allowing potential illness or disease to manifest. Not only is the thought of elements from our bowel movements in our glands and tissues an unattractive thought, it's pretty incredible to think our digestive system was designed to prevent this from happening to us.

Second Brain

Our gut is often referred to as our second brain. There is constant interaction between the gut and the brain. And sometimes the gut is actually the boss of the two. The more we research gut health, the more we see its major impact on mental health. Statistics verify there are a large number of people struggling with anxiety, depression, and panic attacks who are prescribed anti-depressants and anti-anxiety drugs with little hope for improvement. They are also likely told it's genetic and will have to live with it for life. In reality, there *is* hope.

With research and scientific studies supporting the connection between gut and mental health, we need to be looking at gut health. While we don't have the time to get into a lengthy discussion on what is becoming one of my favorite topics to study in relation to this area, please note that, in addition to microbiome communication, there is a major link between our mental health and the vagus nerve. This nerve is part of the parasympathetic nervous system or our "rest and digest" system; it is the longest cranial nerve in the human body that runs from our hairline, through the neck, chest, and out to wrap around almost every major organ in our body *including* nerves that branch out to our gut. This vagus nerve stimulation can be helpful for conditions such as autism, memory disorders, anxiety, migraines, fibromyalgia, tinnitus, and many other conditions in the body. It's involved with neuron receptors, secreting chemicals that control our digestion, our heart rate, our breathing, and our stimulation of hormones. Now how could this *not* have a direct link to our emotions as well as potentially many other health conditions? According to the April 2008 edition of *Science Daily*, BioMed Central states that our diet, inflammation, medical treatments such as chemotherapy, and heavy metals can damage the myelin sheath (the protective coating) on all nerves including the vagus nerve. Therefore, if we focus on reducing our toxins, eating healthy to avoid damage and inflammation, and supplying the body with healing foods and supplements, it may be possible to improve vagus nerve health and thus, our mental health. Depression is a symptom, not a disease. One way to help this symptom is caring for our digestive health.

There you have it. Some key digestive system functions. Functions and interactions your gut performs day in-day out, year after year after year. These functions are extremely hard work and it requires us to have a healthy digestive system if these functions are to be performed properly. If our idea for support is a burger, fries, and diet soda, we are sorely mistaken. Poor diet is a key factor in disrupting gut health. Add in our high-stress lifestyles and toxin bombardment, and we truly have created the perfect storm for body health.

Our Health, Our Choice

Rather than buying into the "it's in our genetics" theory, suppose we have a poor diet and damaged digestive system that is just plain old exhausted and stressed beyond its abilities to function correctly. This is not to say genetics do not affect our health. However, we do have the ability to influence genetics to a certain degree since gut health and diet can improve or avoid many conditions considered genetic such as diabetes, arthritis, high cholesterol, and colon cancer. We can go the route of accepting genetics and taking our medications, or we can take a hard look at our diet and lifestyle. The latter involves more effort, of course, but offers more hope for long-term improvement with much less synthetic interference.

If we have a compromised or stressed digestive system, we ultimately have a large portion of our body affected. We cannot possibly have this much area stressed and not have ramifications. The digestive system is like a finely tuned machine. Each day we put pounds of substances (food, drinks, medications, and supplements) into our mouths hoping that our bodies will be able to filter friend from foe. Overall, our bodies do an impressive job— even though much of what we put in our mouths was foreign to the environment even one hundred years ago. However, based on skyrocketing statistics and the number of doctor visits per year for gut issues, our digestive system is slowly losing the battle. Therefore, *we* are losing the battle...

Do gut issues affect the average person? You can bet they most certainly do. The following two examples are only the tip of the iceberg on the gut's powerful influence and effect:

- Gut issue of IBS (irritable bowel syndrome) alone in 1992 was the second leading cause of missed work, according to The Inside Tract® newsletter from October 2005. If you are an employer who wants to increase work attendance rates, you might want to consider a class for your workforce on gut health. At the very least, hand employees this book to read.

- The digestive system is home to more cancers and causes more cancer mortalities than any other organ system in the body according to Joseph Castro's 2013 article, "11 Surprising Facts About the Digestive System."

As you can see, gut issues do affect the average person. Whether he or she knows it's their gut potentially causing the problem or not is another issue. In the next chapter, we will discuss four key actions to begin supporting and repairing your digestive system.

Chapter Four: The Focus Four

Our very first mission is to soothe and heal the digestive system to aid in soothing inflammation of the entire body. The following is my go-to list of what I like to call the Focus Four. I encourage you to refer back to it when you get overwhelmed with information on ways to improve digestive health. It will remind you of the key areas to keep the focus on gut health. Here are our four Rs of gut health:

1. Recharge Digestion: break down our food and get our nutrients
2. Repair Gut Lining: heal and maintain our digestive system lining to keep toxins out of the bloodstream and avoid inflammation
3. Restore Bacteria and Microbiome Balance: support immunity and nervous system health
4. Rid Toxins and Elimination: keep things moving to get those toxins out of the body

By no means is the Focus Four an exhaustive list for total digestion support. However, most specific gut issues will likely fall under one of these general areas. We will focus on these four tasks, which will very likely improve any other digestive issue and thus, improve overall health. I'll expand slightly on each of the Focus Four before explaining why they are so essential. This is the "important stuff" of our entire body health so hang with me awhile longer!

Recharge Digestion

Many of us possess a pretty sluggish ability to digest our food. A key function of our digestive system is to break down the food we ingest to get the nutrition we need. Digestion literally is hard work on the system and body. It's one reason we tend to get tired after we eat, as it has to expend a great deal of energy to break down the food. Ideally, it does this through its own natural digestive enzymes and also with enzymes in some of the foods we eat (think greens or fruits). However, I could eat three huge green salads per day (actually this many raw veggies all at once can be a burden on a struggling gut), but if the salads do not get broken down within the digestive system, I'm wasting time, energy, fabulous food, and money. Food must be broken down to if we are going to get the benefits it was designed to give. This is one reason some healthy eaters can't seem to make headway on their health issues. A system in need of repair cannot do its job of extracting nutrients from our food. Not only that, a poor-functioning digestive system can result in food that sits in the gut to putrefy, causing acid reflux, bloating, pain, and damage to the lining. Therefore, we must and will discuss support to the system with digestive enzyme supplements and foods and liquids containing natural enzymes.

Repair Gut Lining

In the beginning of our discussion on gut health, we discussed avoiding damaging foods. However, we can't just avoid the damaging foods. It's vital we work on healing past damage and avoid continuing damage to soothe our very precious digestive system lining. You've likely heard the term leaky gut. This term applies to a damaged or compromised gut lining, which is something almost every single one of us has to some degree. A healthy lining secrete enzymes to break down food plus keeps toxins, parasites, and bad bacteria contained in the digestive system so that they eventually are excreted. *A compromised lining cannot do its job.* Thus, the bad guys permeate through this lining that was initially meant to protect us. Toxins permeate into the bloodstream, into our glands, organs, joints, and cells where they do not belong, causing inflammation in these susceptible areas. The problem is, we don't always know inflammation is what's behind our health condition. When we hurt or have some type of autoimmune condition, we assume it's a lifelong malady with no cure or relief.

Restore Bacteria Balance

We are teeming with bacteria. The human body is chock-full of these little fellas—both bad and good—within and *on* the body. Many tend to think of bacteria as a negative, but nothing could be further from the truth. Microbes living in our bodies aren't just there for the ride; they're actively contributing to the normal interactions of the human body. Did you know bacteria balance affects our mood, our skin health, digestive health, our brain health—it's literally a factor in all body systems. We need bacteria for our very existence as well as our immunity. However, what we need is a *balance.* When that microbiome and bacteria balance is compromised with today's diet and culture of sugar, meds, stress, GMOs, and chemicals, we ultimately end up with immunity issues, illness and infections. Then what happens? We use a med or antibiotic to hopefully feel better. But this throws the bacteria and microbiome balance even more out of balance, resulting in further compromised immunity. We end up sick with more antibiotics, which further compromises our microbiome. And the pattern continues. The balance of good *and* bad is vitally important and, actually, having some of the bad bacteria and microbiome is an important contributor to balance as well. What happens to those struggling with health conditions is often a major bacteria imbalance that has set in over time, causing them to have conditions that would seem like they have no connection whatsoever to gut health.

Rid Toxins and Elimination

If we tend toward constipation or irregularity, we consider it inconvenient and sometimes quite uncomfortable. But infrequent bowel movements are so much more than being uncomfortable. Remember those toxins, chemicals, bacteria, and parasites we hope stay within the digestive lining? They should end up in the colon where they eventually leave the body through elimination. If we don't eliminate, we don't remove the toxins and guess where they end up? They hang out for a period of time and eventually absorb back into the body and bloodstream. This creates stress on all body systems by causing an overload of toxins within the body. Even worse, while the toxins didn't leave the body, we've been adding in new ones every single day. The burden on our body systems can be high. While diarrhea is surely the opposite of constipation, it has its own set of issues and is an indication of an upset system making it every bit as bad as constipation. The takeaway on this subject is we *need* regular elimination with normal soft, snakelike stools.

If each of us turned to our gut health to begin working on overall body health, we could potentially save time, energy and frustration while possibly avoiding the need to treat other symptoms and areas of the body that are the end result of the inflammation that begins in the gut. If we treat the symptoms but the inflamed digestive system remains, the issues will remain or intensify.

As we ease and soothe inflammation, we remove stress on the body. You'd be amazed how the body can kick in with its inherent, natural ability to heal when given an optimum environment. Ideally, the process goes as follows:

- We heal (and support) the digestive system.
- This removes the bombardment of toxins and inflammation filtrating into the bloodstream.
- This takes stress off the symptomatic and inflamed body parts (joints, brain, colon, thyroid).
- The affected body parts get a break from being attacked or inflamed and the body's natural healing can begin.

When all goes well, healing begins without medications, which may actually interfere with this ability to heal.

Keep in mind that even though the body is amazing in its ability to repair and rebound, it may take some time to feel change. It won't happen in just a few weeks. It is an ongoing process where some days are two steps forward, and some days 1.5 steps back. But that's OK because you are still making progress!

I will be listing ways we can support the digestive system at the end of each section. While I will mention supplements, I also remind you that we may want to avoid going overboard on them. If we change our diet plus ease our stress and toxins so we offer support to the system, that's every bit as important as supplements. There are a few supplements I consider must-haves, and I will emphasize them. But, overall, the most important thing you can do is search out organic, whole food and eat lots of it. Real food is where the best nutrients and support will come.

Let's now expand on each of the Rs in the Focus Four to see what we can (and need) to do to help support this hard-working digestive system of ours.

Chapter Five: Recharge Digestion

Recharging digestion is pretty important stuff and the reason it is first on the Focus Four list. It's also the first step in the digestive system process. If we don't get this first step covered, we can't possibly expect the following digestive processes to be functioning correctly.

We begin with the topic of digestion because when we digest our food, if all goes well, we are literally breaking it down into minute particles to extract nutrients from the food-no small task but vital to good health!

Components of an optimal digestive system:

- Breaks down food to extract nutrients
- Nutrients absorb and pass into the bloodstream
- Body systems are supported with the nutrients provided from the nutrients delivered

Pretty simple, right?

Simple technically, but in reality the majority of us have our food sitting in our gut like a big, rotting lump. Many are *not* getting food broken down; thus, they do not digest. Therefore, the vital nutrients from our food are not getting absorbed. The body *cannot* secrete proper hormones, move our legs, think clearly, give us energy, good metabolism for proper weight, and perform our daily functions if it doesn't get the nutrients it needs from our food. Nothing could be more basic and important yet it's a vastly overlooked problem in our healthcare system. To get the nutrients means the food must, must, must digest; it *must* go from pieces of food that enter the stomach to a micro particle that can be absorbed. What process accomplishes this? Digestion—the process of breaking down food.

Many of us invest in high-quality supplements like vitamins or minerals; yet, we are unaware of the value and need of things like getting our nutrients from our foods through digestive enzymes. This is rather like putting the cart before the horse. We zero in on what vitamin to buy and use yet have no emphasis on getting that same nutrient naturally through the process of digestion. Vitamins are fine, but they are a supplement to the vitamins and nutrients we might not be extracting from the most natural and effective source on this earth—our food!

I read a recent study from www.livescience.com, in which author Christopher Wanjek announced the discovery that low B12 was a factor in aging, autism, and schizophrenia (February 2016). Thus, the study was recommending supplements of B12. I have no doubt B12 supplementation is super important for the body, but in almost all of these studies on low B12, low zinc, low niacin, or any other important vitamin, the recommendation is often to add that particular supplement to your daily protocol. Yes, adding it can be helpful, but let's also recommend digestion as it's very likely people with these conditions either aren't eating the foods containing that vitamin or, just as possible, they may be eating the food but not getting the nutrients extracted through digestion. It would be better to recommend including digestive enzymes in order to *get* the nutrients with the inclusion of the needed vitamin or mineral. We can't put the focus on ingesting a supplement more than eating correct foods and breaking down the food in the body.

Do not underestimate the work involved and the burden put on our stomachs to digest food. This means the system needs to take that chunk of food coming down the chute and must literally dissolve or break it down into an absorbable micro particle.

The Problems of Inadequate Enzymes

What can happen in the body if we don't have enough of our own enzymes or don't use supplemental digestive enzymes, resulting in suboptimal digestion? It's not just a matter of wasting good food. If we don't digest our food properly, it really has no choice but to hang out in our stomach like a guest overstaying its welcome. This is the vicious health cycle involved in poor digestion:

1. Inadequate enzymes cause food to sit undigested in the stomach, resulting in the body sensing a problem of not enough acid or enzymes.

2. The brain receives the signals that there is a problem of undigested food sitting in the stomach and sends out an SOS for the need of enzymes. This leads to the body sending an overabundance of acid and enzymes to compensate.

3. The overabundance of enzymes and acid causes burning and pain in the stomach and throat.

4. The overabundance of enzymes and acid causes damage to the digestive lining.

5. This person struggling now uses an over-the-counter (OTC) heartburn tablet or a prescription med to block stomach acid and enzymes.

6. The person now has *less* stomach acid and *fewer* enzymes to break down his next meal, which can mean less absorption of nutrients and another cycle of excess enzymes and acid being sent it.

7. The medications used for the heartburn and excess acid interfere with natural enzymes and can compromise the stomach lining even further, creating an infiltration of toxins into the bloodstream.

8. The infiltration of toxins leads to inflammation, which causes a myriad of health issues that require medications.

9. The medications cause more potential stomach lining damage, which leads to even less natural enzymes and acids for breaking down food.

Where did all this begin? With low stomach acid from an unhealthy digestive system leading to undigested food leading to the body overreacting with excess enzymes. This results in heartburn or acid reflux that led to medications rather than using digestive enzymes or natural alternatives such as apple cider vinegar to help the stomach digest foods.

This health cycle that begins with the very first step of not digesting our food causes a long list of potential health issues. (Note, this is only the list for the process of "digest" or breaking down of food. The list for potential issues for the entire digestive system is much longer.) They potential issues from lack of digestion include:

- Acid and Burning: It's labor-intensive work for the gut to break down the food we eat. Ideally, we have enough of our own stomach acids and enzymes to dissolve it. However, the majority of the population has a compromised digestive system and does not produce enough natural enzymes and acids. If we don't break down the food, it remains a chunk in the stomach and putrefies. As we previously discussed, the system senses a problem then kicks into overdrive to send not only adequate enzymes but also extra hydrochloric acid (HCL) in an attempt to get it out of the stomach. This can result in too much stomach acid. Now, we have burning or acid reflux. Thus, ironically, stomach acid many times can be caused by too little enzymes and acid in the initial phase of digestion rather than too much. However, if you visit the doctor's office or listen to the commercials, you are advised to block the production of stomach acid and to take one of the leading prescriptions and over-the-counter meds. What will this ultimately do? It will cause even more problems breaking down food and get you even fewer nutrients. Ironically, it more likely we actually need *more* acid and enzymes to break down the food at the beginning of the digestive process in the first place.

- Bloating: This can happen when food does not break down in the stomach. Undigested food putrefies, creating gas and resulting in a large or swollen belly as well as gas that does not have enough escape routes.

- Pain: Just like any other damaged body part, when the gut malfunctions and has to work overtime to do its job, it hurts!

- Burping: Like bloating, burping can happen when food does not break down in the stomach rather than digesting. Undigested food putrefies, creating gas.

- Gas: If people don't want to stand by you, you can't blame them. This is a stinky problem and goes along the same line as bloating and burping. We need to break down our food to get it out of our belly!

- Inadequate Nutrient Absorption: The stomach is supposed to produce enough hydrochloric acid and enzymes to break down our food extracting and delivering the nutrients from the food to our body. When we don't break down food, the nutrients aren't extracted and can't be delivered. You can eat the healthiest foods in the world, but if your gut does not break down the food so the nutrients can be released, your body can't thrive, regenerate, and repair. Once again, this helps explain why some people say, "I'm a super healthy eater. Why don't I feel better?"

• Small Intestinal Bacteria Overgrowth (SIBO): Optimal levels of stomach acids and enzymes help keep bacteria overgrowth in check. Your digestive system environment—when functioning properly—is designed to keep bacteria and parasites in line. If that environment doesn't have the enzymes to keep them under control, these guys get to have a party (with *you* as the host) in not only your gut but throughout the bloodstream. Before ever venturing on a parasite or candida cleanse, it would be vital to get the gut environment in tip-top shape with enzymes and HCL digesting your food (along with gut repair that we will discuss in an upcoming section). If you don't, your cleanse may initially clear out the bad guys. However, if even a few remain or are reintroduced to the body but we haven't built the proper level of acid to create an unwelcome environment, they will start the party all over again. Think of your digestive enzymes as the party poopers for the bad guys.

Every time we put *any* food or liquid in our system, many processes need to interact to break it down. Breaking down food and sorting the nutrients from the waste is an intensive process for the digestive system. If the system is in good shape, all is well. However, if it is compromised, all is *far* from well. I compare a compromised digestive system to trying to run a mile with an injured knee. It's difficult, right? As you favor the injured knee, it puts stress on your back, your hips, your foot, and even the uninjured knee. Pretty soon, these parts also start to hurt and put stress on additional body parts. The end result is a body with many tired, stressed or damaged body parts that all originated from the injured knee and continued stress from not resting the knee. The same applies to our gut. When it's functioning properly, it helps all other body parts function properly. When it is damaged or compromised, it's much more difficult to break down anything we eat or drink. Other parts of the body (glands, organs, muscles, joints, etc.) will end up stressed as well, and your most susceptible area will feel the effects first. Thyroid gland issues? Arthritis? Anxiety? Consider poor digestion for these and many other health issues as a possible culprit!

Support to Digest

Now that we understand the importance of helping our digestive system digest our food, what are some specific ways we can help it with this hard work? Here are some important actions you can take to help digest:

- Avoid stress near mealtime as much as possible.
- Chew (and chew and chew and chew) your food.
- Use digestive enzymes supplements. (These are vastly different than probiotics so don't confuse the two.)
- Eat or drink certain foods to help aid the digestion process.

Let's expand a little on each of these digestion helpers.

Avoid Stress Near Mealtime

To ease or remove stress is an important part of helping your digestion break down your food. Stress creates high cortisol, fast heartbeat, and limited blood flow to the stomach, which can completely interfere with much of the digestive system. Think fight or flight. The body stops or slows down everything to prepare the body for flight. This includes digestion. When we slow down digestion (or have it come to a complete halt), we will not receive our last meal's nutrients, and we likely caused damage to the system through undigested food resulting in excess acid. If you are not in a good place mentally when you sit down to eat, get up and walk away until you are.

Sometimes we just can't change the cause of our stress (finances, spouse, children, relatives, employer, illness, etc.), so we must find avenues to help us with how we react to it. We will discuss stress-reducing activities, such as prayer, meditation, yoga, and structured breathing prior to the meal, in more detail in a later chapter.

Chew your Food

Another digestion helper is thoroughly chewing your food. Remember, the stomach has no teeth! The dilemma of escalating gut health statistics is somewhat explainable just from the simple process of inadequate chewing. Look around when you go to a restaurant and observe how the average person eats. Watch how fast they eat and how hard they have to swallow. If we have to swallow hard, we aren't chewing enough. Many times, we think the stomach solely breaks down food when actually an important part of digestion begins in the mouth with salivary enzymes and mouth action. This action partially liquefies as well as breaks the food into more tolerable sizes for the stomach to begin its job of breaking down our food to the microscopically small pieces needed for nutrient absorption. Dine, don't gulp. Remember it's a big task for the stomach to break down your food. It needs help! Chewing is a great way to increase your odds of getting your nutrients and avoiding a lump of food damaging the gut. As a bonus, thoroughly chewing takes you longer to eat so that you have time for the brain to signal when you are full without overeating. This means chewing more could be your new weight-loss plan! What else can we do to help digest our food?

Use Digestive Enzymes

If I had to choose only two supplements for my entire body—not just the digestive system—it would be probiotics and digestive enzymes. There tends to be confusion that these are one and the same. I've had people tell me they don't need digestive enzymes because they take a good probiotic. The two are very different, and both are extremely important. We will talk about probiotics and why they are vital farther into this chapter on digestive health but for now, let's focus on enzymes. The message I would love to get across to every single person on this earth would be the necessity of considering digestive enzyme supplements as a key helper in the digestion process.

It used to be that naturopaths and health advisors would say almost all adults over age twenty-five do not make or have adequate natural enzymes. However, in today's world of processed food, stress, gluten, and GMOs, almost every single adult, most teens, and even children can be lacking in natural enzymes and acid. Again, you won't necessarily have obvious symptoms, but the risk of irritation, inflammation, and lack of nutrients is too great not to consider supplementation of enzymes. Insufficient stomach acid leads to a stressed digestive system *and* a lack of nutrient absorption that can reflect not only in health issues but also on your outward appearance. If you are concerned about the cost for enzymes, replace spending money at the beauty counter with getting digestive enzymes. You'll be money (and looks) ahead in the long run.

The array of digestive enzymes offered on the shelves or Internet today can be confusing, causing some who have made the (wise) decision to supplement with enzymes to get overwhelmed and give up. Don't give up; don't walk away. I would recommend you avoid the cheap drugstore or big box store brands. Some great brands are ReNew Life, Pure, Dr. Mercola, and Dr. Axe. For now, as long as it's from a company that specializes in supplements, you should be good to go. Some companies include probiotics in the digestive enzymes complex; there is some digestive benefit with probiotics, but it likely won't be enough probiotic to replace the need for a separate probiotic supplement.

As you get started using your digestive enzymes, you can always expand into researching if one brand or type is your preference over another but, for now, just pick one so you avoid the pitfall of being overwhelmed causing inaction. I'll explain a few different types of enzymes below, but again, if in doubt, just get a bottle of your basic digestive enzymes to get started. Here are a few different types of enzymes you might see when you're shopping:

Digestive Enzymes

These are your basic needs. Listed on the bottle, you will see things like Bromelain, Papaya, Pepsin, Pectin, Licorice, Amylase, Glucoamylase, Lipase, Pancreatin, Protease, Invertase, Maltase, Cellulase, Bromelain, Turmeric, Fennel, Peppermint, and Lactase. I like to use digestive enzymes at the beginning of the meal, but check the directions on the bottle.

Betaine HCL or Digestive Enzymes with HCL

Some enzyme formulations have Betaine HCL in them. HCL is hydrochloric acid. This is something our digestive system should make naturally, but as we discussed, almost all of us do not make enough due a damaged system. HCL is best for helping break down the heavy-duty stuff like meats, eggs, and other proteins. If you eat mostly vegetables and starches, you may not need as much HCL. For heavy meals, I like to use digestive enzymes *with HCL,* and for snacks or light meals that don't have the heavy protein, I use the digestive enzymes without HCL. You may need more than one capsule per meal, but if you feel burning when you use your HCL, back off on the amount you use. Follow package directions. Those with stomach ulcers should not supplement with HCL.

Bile Salts

While these are not necessarily for everybody, if you have had your gallbladder removed you very likely really need bile salts in addition to your digestive enzymes. You can find these at a good health food store or on the Internet.

Proteolytic Enzymes

This type of enzyme is normally used in the morning before eating and at night before bed for cleansing of the blood, support to the immune system, improved circulation, etc. While these can be great additions to your enzyme protocol, the focus at first, in my opinion, needs to be your digestive enzymes and HCL to break down food. You can surely also use proteolytic enzymes, but if you are concerned with trying to remember what to take and when, focus on digestive enzymes for now and consider proteolytic enzymes when you are ready to add them to your daily regimen.

Pancreatic Enzymes

These enzymes are normally included in a good digestive enzyme supplement. If you have had pancreas issues, it may be worth adding in a booster with a separate bottle of pancreatic enzymes.

With digestive enzymes and HCL, the usage directions might instruct you to use one with each meal. Honestly, that may not be nearly enough, especially those of us struggling with gut health leading to inadequate natural enzyme production. A good way to find how many you need is to add one additional capsule with each normal-size meal. Start with one capsule per meal, increase to two, then three until you feel a slight burning. When that happens, back down to the last number you took that didn't burn. For me, I was up to seven with each meal. I know that's a lot, and you may not need that much, but, then again, you may. As you help ease stress on the gut with supplemental enzymes, it can begin its healing process and, over time, you should eventually be able to back off on the amount of enzymes you supplement.

There are people who believe using digestive enzymes leads the body to rely on the supplement rather than producing enzymes on its own. I respect that opinion, and I'm certainly all for reducing supplements where we can, but I also believe that almost every person in America is lacking natural enzymes due to the standard American diet. Lacking enzymes places stress on the digestive system and leads to damage, which is a bigger risk than the outside chance enzyme supplements might deplete your natural enzyme production.

The goal right now, however, is to take the burden off the system so it *can* heal and, of course, break down your food. I would honestly never back down to zero because, again, most all of us need at least 1-2 supplements with meals. I see pretty much zero negatives and a whole lot of benefits come from taking these enzymes. If you are feeling better, eating right, and experiencing no burning, I advise to keep the digestive enzyme supplement going.

Using digestive enzymes with meals will hopefully become a habit for you each time you eat. I keep some in my purse and even when I eat out, make sure to use them. They do no good if they don't get used. The same applies to eating at home. It's a rare meal that I don't use my digestive enzyme supplements, and I recommend the same to you.

Eat or Drink Certain Foods

In addition to digestive enzyme supplements, you can also eat certain foods or drink to help get the digestive juices/enzymes flowing. This should *not* be in place of enzymes supplements-at least until your system is in great shape- but in addition to them. Foods or drinks to help get digestive enzymes flowing to aid in the process of breaking down our food:

Organic Apple Cider Vinegar (ACV)

ACV is a perfect example of Mother Nature providing us what we need. It supports our natural enzyme production process as well as being alkaline forming to help neutralize body PH and prevent acid. You can start with using a teaspoon and work up to a tablespoon if needed. Find what works for you. Start out with this small amount at first since using more can be "too much too fast" and bother some people's stomach. If it bothers, don't stop-use less. I use it first thing in the morning to help with PH balance, which helps with stomach environment. If it bothers your stomach, wait until you have a little food with eventually using it in water five minutes before meals (unless it bothers your empty stomach) to help get your digestive juices flowing. It's best if you don't drink it in a big glass of water, as too much liquid prior to a meal is not recommended. Your bottle of ACV should say "with the mother" if it's going to be helpful to digestion. The mother is the dark, cloudy substance in the ACV formed from naturally occurring pectin and apple residues; it appears as molecules of protein connected in strand-like chains. The presence of the mother shows that the best part of the apple has not been destroyed. Vinegars containing the mother have enzymes and minerals that other vinegars may not contain due to over-processing, filtration, and overheating. It also makes for a refreshing "pick me up" midday, replacing that damaging soda some like to have. It's a good idea to swish a small amount of water in your mouth after drinking the ACV to remove it from your teeth. While it's good for the stomach, it's not so good for tooth enamel.

Matcha Tea

This is the powerhouse of teas. It's high in antioxidants, but for our purposes in this section, what's highly important is that it promotes intestinal regularity and a healthy digestive system. It comes in pulverized, loose-leaf form. Therefore, there could be a few floaters or residue at the bottom of the cup, but that's OK! It's also rich in fiber, chlorophyll, and vitamins. Even if you aren't a tea drinker, it's worth having a cup of this now and then. Be sure the brand you use is organic. I use Kenko Tea Matcha Green and purchase it through Amazon. It's a tad pricey, but you use a tiny amount per cup to do the job so it lasts a long time.

Lemon

Lemon in your water isn't just to make it taste good; it's also great for getting those taste buds revved up (think sour!) which naturally tells the brain and gut to start getting those digestive juices going. It's also important for body PH so that excess stomach acid might be neutralized. If you tend to burn in the tummy or throat, squeeze some lemon in your water to help reduce the irritation.

Soup

For centuries, soup was served at the beginning of the meal. There's a reason! Soup is normally lighter fare so the digestive system gets informed there's food coming down the hatch. The ingredients in many kinds of soups get the natural digestive enzymes ready for the heavier food yet to come, and that's a good thing.

Salad

Like soup, there's a reason salad is also served at the beginning of a meal to help with digestion. It's normally a tad easier to break down, and it introduces food to the digestive system prior to the heavier foods yet to come so we get those digestive juices flowing. In addition, the raw vegetables will have natural enzymes to help break down the upcoming meal. We are talking mainly about a lighter salad in this case. If you are having a big chef salad or some other large salad, then I like to get my digestive enzymes supplement down with it. Even though vegetables (and fruit) do have natural enzymes, a large salad also has a lot of fiber and other items that take work to break down. Unfortunately, many restaurants are now skipping the soup or salad, as it's not as popular in America as with other cultures. Americans have a bad habit of bolting down food and moving on to the next thing in their lives. Slow down, eat your soup or salad, and then enjoy your meal. Your digestive system will thank you.

Fennel Seeds

Some cultures chew on fennel seeds after a meal to help cleanse the palate, but like most practices used by other cultures, it also serves another purpose. It helps digestive enzymes break down our food.

Fresh Ginger

Grate this into your drinking water, tea, over your salad, etc. Ginger is great for not only soothing the tummy but also helping with digestion.

Black Pepper

This hasn't been on tables since ancient times only for flavor. Black pepper can work with your digestive juices to help absorb nutrients. Anything that helps absorb nutrients is a *must* in my world. Ideally, avoid the stuff at the big box stores, and look at the health section of your grocery store for pepper grinders with the peppercorns in it. This makes for a little fresher, purer pepper. If you're an essential oil person like me, you could add a drop or two of high-quality oil that can be ingested at the end of cooking. (Otherwise, you cook out any benefit of the oil.) One of my favorite ways to use my oil is in my bone broth after I've heated it up.

I've always been a salt girl and truthfully felt no need for the spice of pepper. It didn't bother me; I just didn't add it. As I learn more on black pepper and its ability to help absorb nutrients, I have started using it regularly and recommend you do as well. Turns out, it's not spicy hot (in my opinion), has great flavor, *and* helps with nutrient absorption. Cool stuff!

<u>Sea Salt or Himalayan Salt</u>

Just like pepper, there's a reason salt is normally on every table. It's another great digestive aid. However, please avoid the common table salt, which is pretty much crap. It has normally been bleached, processed, and stripped of any mineral value. When doctors advise against salt, you can bet they should be referring to common table salt. Unless you have kidney issues or unless your doctor has some good reason to advise against them, you should benefit from real sea salt or Himalayan salt since they contain minerals without the bleaching process of table salt. Salt activates enzymes needed for proper digestive processes and is required by the parietal cells of the stomach wall to make hydrochloric acid.

We're far better off to change our diet to assist in providing enzymes through our food that can help extract the nutrients from the food. A vitamin or mineral supplement while good is just that a *supplement*. It cannot possibly replace the interaction of the constituents in each food to help us absorb and provide nutrients from real food. Thus, we should supplement with enzymes in addition to *not* instead of real food.

The topics we just discussed are by no means a comprehensive list. Avoiding stress, chewing our food, taking digestive enzymes, and eating foods—all practices that help with digestion—are great ways to get started helping our gut. You don't need to do everything right off the bat, but you surely should get going on doing some of them. Pick one or two and incorporate them into your daily routine for a week or two before adding others. More importantly than doing it all is doing it consistently. I have listed a beginner's list for supporting the entire digestive system at the end of this chapter. Start there. Add from the lists at the end of each section on the Focus Four as you develop good additions and habits.

If you don't remember anything else from this chapter on digestion, try to recall digestive enzymes. This will be a great place to start (and continue) to get at least some of the burden off that overworked gut.

Sum It Up

We *digest* to break down food into micro particles more easily absorbed into the bloodstream to get our nutrients. We *digest* to avoid chunks of food in the stomach that irritate and cause damage to the stomach lining. And, we digest to separate the "good from the bad" as far as nutrients vs toxins. To properly digest, we must:

- Avoid stress at all times but especially near mealtime.
- Chew your food. Dine rather than gulp.
- Ease the burden on your system by using digestive enzymes supplements with meals.
- Eat or drink certain foods to help heal *and* aid in your natural digestive enzymes process.

There we have it. A good start on helping our gut do the hard work of digestion to relieve some stress and allow it to heal. Before moving on to anything else, start with this list and begin taking the stress off not only the digestive system, but ultimately, the entire body.

Now give yourself a great big pat on the back! You just finished the first of the Focus Four list. Don't feel exhausted thinking you've only learned one of the Focus Four. The other three steps make more sense, having learned why it's important to digest for proper digestion; plus, many of the foods and habits in this chapter are the same for the remaining three Rs of: Repair gut lining, Restore proper microbiome balance, and Rid toxins.

Cheat Sheet to Recharge Digestion-Digest Your Food!

Ease Stress	-NOT-	Hurried Lifestyle
• Prayer, mediation, quiet time prior to meals		• Eating while working, upset, rushed

Rest the Gut	-NOT-	Stress on the Gut
• Chew, chew, chew		• Gulping and inhaling
• Lighter, more frequent meals		• Heavy meals in one sitting
• Soup		• Meat
• Salad		• Potatoes

Supplement to Help Digest	-NOT-	Supplements Hampering Digestion
• Digestive enzymes		• Medications that block natural enzymes and acid
• HCL (hydrochloric acid) with meats and protein		• Using no enzymes to aid digestion
• Bile salts (for those with gallbladder issues)		
• Pancreatic enzymes (for those with pancreas issues)		

Helpful Drinks & Seasonings	-NOT-	Damaging Drinks & Seasonings
• Apple Cider Vinegar		• Alcohol
• Lemon in water		• Caffeine
• Fennel		• Soda

- Black Pepper

- Himalayan and Sea Salt

- Ginger, Anise, Tarragon

- Matcha Tea

- Processed table salt

Chapter Six: Repair Gut Lining

Now that we fully understand the importance of proper digestion, let's move on to the step two on our list to achieving and maintaining a healthy gut. As a reminder of our goal, here is the Focus Four of gut health:

1. Recharge Digestion: break down our food and get our nutrients

2. Repair Gut Lining: heal and maintain the digestive system lining and keep toxins out of bloodstream to help avoid inflammation

3. Restore Bacteria and Microbiome Balance: support our immunity and nervous system health

4. Rid Toxins and Elimination: poop to get those toxins out of the body

We have completed the discussion of the first step on the list-recharge to digest. In step two, repair gut lining, I hope to convey the impact of a damaged gut lining on your overall health as well as the steps you can take for repair. You have nothing to lose and potentially so much to gain by taking the time to learn about a damaged gut lining-commonly known as "leaky gut".

Here are just a few reasons you should be concerned with leaky gut:

- Damaging foods and habits erode the lining of our digestive system.

- A damaged lining develops "holes" that allows toxins and invaders to travel outside the digestive system into the bloodstream.

- These toxins do not belong in the bloodstream and are highly inflammatory.
- Inflamed glands, joints, muscles, as well as the entire body, *will* have pain and disruption of their normal function.

We call a compromised digestive lining (and thus, a compromised digestive system) leaky gut. Leaky gut is something many naturopaths, nutritionists, and chiropractors discuss as the starting point of good health. (Another reason I always trust my natural health community more than western medicine.)

We are finally beginning to see a flood of research from the medical community to verify leaky gut exists even though they failed to acknowledge this potential problem for years and dismissed its significance to overall body health. With that, leaky gut is being given a technical medical name called 'intestinal permeability'. Knowing how pharmaceutical companies work, it probably won't be long before there will be some type of pill/medicine created to "help" with leaky gut. But you should know, there will never, *ever* be a pill that will heal a leaky gut all by itself. Healing involves a myriad of processes that need to happen (requiring our active involvement). One thing alone will never do it. The superb news on leaky gut is by helping it heal, you help *you* heal.

Leaky Gut

We will discuss leaky gut *but* to fully comprehend the impact of its damage, it's important to review the size of the entire digestive system, not only the stomach. The digestive system includes the roof of the mouth, down the esophagus, through the stomach, small and large intestines, colon, and rectum. As I've previously mentioned, it encompasses roughly the square feet of one full tennis court. That's a heck of a lot of distance in the body! Now keep in mind that *all* of this is lined with a protective mucosal lining (kind of like the protective slime on the outside of a fish) that, once compromised, is no longer protective. When this happens, it becomes something referred to as leaky gut.

Your entire digestive tract is lined with this protective mucosal lining that acts as a net with extremely small holes (like a sieve or strainer). The lining is made up of bacteria and microbiome with neuron receptors that allow only specific substances like properly digested food, nutrients, vitamins, and enzymes to pass through and into the bloodstream.

With a well-functioning digestive system, this protective net keeps toxins, viruses, bacteria, parasites, and pathogens contained within the digestive system and isolated from the bloodstream. These toxins are ideally contained within the digestive system and properly excreted from the body through the process of elimination. The bacteria as they naturally exist within the digestive tract are perfectly harmless and beneficial, helping digestion and absorption of food. However, when these bacteria enter the body and the blood, they become harmful, inflammatory, and damaging.

If we have leaky gut, it indicates our protective mucosal lining of the digestive system is losing some of its protective capabilities as stress, foods, and chemicals damage it; this causes holes for toxins to escape into the body. No wonder it's called leaky gut! Although this is not a pretty thought, consider how your poop smells. Poop or waste is comprised of the "bad stuff" your digestive system, in its amazing ability, sorts out from your food and drink. This smelly, toxic waste *should* leave our body as undesirable and unneeded waste product. Now imagine it doesn't leave your body but rather, recirculates through your body. The toxins, bacteria, parasites, pathogens, and viruses act like little worms, making their way through the holes caused by damage in the digestive lining. These toxins are now in your bloodstream to be delivered in a damaging form to your cells, glands, tissues, nerve myelin sheath, and organs instead of going out in your poop.

Toxins in the bloodstream being delivered to every corner of the body equate to major inflammation in the body. These do not belong anywhere in the body, which is why the digestive system, in its miraculous design, is supposed to rid them from our body. Unfortunately, stress, chemicals, our standard diets, *and* our poor excuse for a food supply only add fuel to the fire for damaging the mucosal gut lining.

Many times, our most susceptible area of the body will be the first affected from inflammation and toxins delivered to that area through leaky gut. Each of us is different and so are the issues that arise. The average person does tend to have some of these susceptible areas in common such as thyroid, joints, skin health, nerve health, and even mental health conditions like anxiety and depression. However, these are far from the only potential areas affected. This is important for those with common health issues but even more so for those with autoimmune conditions. Because, ultimately, what *is* an autoimmune condition? An autoimmune condition (arthritis, MS, lupus, arthritis, hair loss, type I diabetes, etc.) is the body attacking its own healthy cells. Actually, the theory behind leaky gut is that the body is not attacking the healthy cell as much as it is attacking the *invader* of the cell—the toxin, bacteria, virus, or pathogen that has been delivered and permeated the cell lining into the cell itself. The body is only doing its job when it is attacking that cell invader.

While western medicine throws prescription medications and even extreme attempts such as chemotherapy treatments or steroid meds to heal autoimmune conditions, they are failing to look at the root cause. Why would our body, in its innate ability to heal and repair, attack its own healthy cells? Our body *is* trying to heal and repair by attacking the invader. It's not normal for these invaders to permeate the cells, but due to leaky gut, the abnormal becomes reality. Because modern medicine does not approach health from a holistic point of view, they do not view leaky gut as a possible factor in autoimmune conditions.

When you consider the description of leaky gut, it makes sense that the body is doing what it does naturally—it's attacking and trying to remove a foreign invader that has permeated a healthy cell. If you've been told your condition is incurable, you might want to take a good hard look at your gut health. If you don't, I would agree with western medicine that these things are incurable. If we bombard an already compromised body with powerful (think toxic) medications or chemo drugs to try to kill the invaders, there's no question the healthy portion of the cell is going to be affected since these drugs surely cannot distinguish healthy from sick. It makes more sense to work on creating an environment that makes it difficult for the invader to ever leave the digestive system by healing the gut lining rather than poisoning or killing your own human cells. As long as we continue to eat with a leaky gut, we continue to allow more toxins into those cells.

By no means is leaky gut only related to autoimmune conditions. If you have leaky gut, it's likely related to all or any of your health conditions at least in some way or another. Many parents of a child with autism have seen their child experience a mood swing after eating a food that irritates. For many of these children, diet change has improved mental health a little for some and greatly for many. This is just one example of how diet, inflammation and the mind connection interact in our body systems.

While I am not claiming any and all health conditions or autoimmune issues will be healed by working on gut health, I am emphasizing the possibilities of the many healing abilities of the body when we repair or maintain gut health so that we no longer have toxic and damaging substances infiltrating through the gut lining and into our bloodstream to be carried throughout the body and brain. Focusing on the root cause is ultimately the key to helping our body do its job of healing. Now that you are aware (or soon will be) of the ramifications of leaky gut, you can help your body repair its gut lining and move down the road to better health.

Healing Leaky Gut

So what can we do to avoid or heal leaky gut? Many of the actions listed here overlap with the list for helping digestion, making it easier to incorporate the following into your daily routine.

- Avoid and/or reduce stress.
- Avoid heavy meals and damaging foods.
- Eat healing, easy-to-digest foods.
- Avoid chemicals and medications.
- Support with supplements.

Avoid and/or Reduce Stress

I cannot overemphasize the damage stress does to the stomach and gut. Working on gut health really does involve working on emotional health at the same time. You may have heard the saying "eats at my gut" when it comes to being upset or nervous. Well, it's true, *and* it's vital to incorporate some practices to help you get stress under control.

This, of course, is so much easier said than done. However, stress can at least be reduced. We can't always control the things that cause our stress, but we can (and must) learn to control how we react to it. I used to put easing stress last on this list of ways to help our digestive system but after years of fighting to get a healthier gut, it finally became clear. I was spinning my wheels if I didn't get my stress under control. Call it what you will—stress, nervousness, anxiety, worry, fear, regret, anger, being rushed all the time, etc. It comes down to the fact that being stressed *will* greatly impact gut health. We will discuss some stress-reduction ideas in an upcoming chapter but, in the meantime, be aware how important it is to reduce stress to improve gut health (and whole body health).

Avoid Heavy Meals and Damaging Foods
Heavy meals to a leaky gut are like hitting a man when he's already down. I cannot overemphasize how much work it is for our digestive system to properly digest a meal. When we quickly inhale our food in one huge meal instead of eating smaller meals slowly, we aren't giving the digestive system a chance. The gut cannot digest fast enough so food sits, putrefies, irritates, and causes lining damage.

Let's look at some of the other contributing factors of leaky gut. Once again, keep in mind that we can use supplements or soothing foods to work on healing, but if we continue to cause damage, we cannot heal. This causes a lot of frustration for many people. They might do the good habits by incorporating bone broth, light meals, and healthy fats or other suggestions but continue their other normal daily habits as usual. They don't necessarily know they are damaging. This would only be 50 percent of the equation. Incorporating the good but continuing the bad will ultimately lead to frustration. We can feel like we're doing these good things for the gut yet not see the healing we want. This can lead to giving up the good habits, thinking they don't help. An attempt can be made, but if we don't remove the damaging habits, foods, and drinks that we will discuss in this chapter, the stress and damage will continue; the body will work overtime to not only repair but also survive the damage.

Popcorn

If you are eating microwave popcorn, you should be aware that the buttery flavor is actually a chemical called diacetyl linked to possible long-term neurological toxicity, according to the University of Minnesota Center for Drug Design's 2012 abstract on butter flavorant. In addition, the lining of the bag has chemicals that are very difficult for the body to break down and eliminate meaning these chemicals remain in the body rather than being excreted. To add to the list of negatives for microwave popcorn, it is very difficult to digest. This popular snack food also interferes with brain health, toxicity, and gut health. This would be an important one to remove from the diet. Although regular popcorn can be difficult to digest, it would be better than microwave popcorn. When I do indulge in regular popcorn, I use my AirPopper, top it with a combo of butter (organic, from grass-fed cows), organic, unrefined coconut oil, and sea salt. I am sure to use digestive enzymes when I eat it. It's a snack I limit because it's still a burden as far as breaking it down to digest but the enzymes help, the butter and coconut oil are good fats plus there are good minerals in the sea salt (and it's yummy!). This makes it a far better choice than microwaved popcorn.

Bread

This is one of the biggest sources of irritation to our gut due to the gluten our modern-day breads contain. Ancient breads contained natural enzymes and probiotics. Therefore, the tummy we evolved with is one that had assistance within the bread itself for getting it digested. But our bread today is not the bread it once was. Our digestive system pretty much doesn't know what to do with this soft (bread was never intended to be soft), gooey, unrecognizable substance. This "substance" sits in the stomach and is very difficult to break down causing stomach lining irritation. Almost all restaurants give you a big basket of bread with the soup or salad served. This will pretty much undo any benefit of the soup or salad since bread is chewy, gluey, and a big *phooey* to the digestive system. More on this subject later but suffice it to say, get that bread off the table!

Nuts

While they have loads of good nutrients, nuts can be tough on the tummy to break down; this equates to stress on the system. If you eat nuts, be sure to follow our practice we just discussed of chewing thoroughly, using enzymes, and limiting the amount so you don't cause an unnecessary burden.

Excessive Alcohol or Coffee

As with everything, moderation is key. Avoid drinking alcohol or coffee on an empty stomach since both are eroding and irritating to the gut lining. I like to put a pinch of baking soda in my coffee to help with the acidity and ease a tad bit of the burden. A spoonful of coconut oil prior to alcohol helps ease the blood sugar spike alcohol causes as well as soothes the tummy.

GMO (genetically modified) and GE (Genetically engineered) Foods

Genetically modified foods are a result of altering the seeds of our plants, which can ultimately cause great damage to the digestive system and whole body. GMO plants are engineered to withstand high amounts of pesticides. This is so the farmer can spray the weeds heavily to eliminate them yet the food plant remains. The theory from the creators of GMOs is that these chemicals break down and no longer reside in the plant by the time it gets to our table. I suspect they have a bridge to sell us as well.

Up to 85 percent of corn in the states is GMO. Therefore, corn and processed (think packaged) food products containing corn oil (which is many) will likely have GMO corn. Sunflowers and soy crops make up a high percentage of GMO and GE plants. Almost any packaged product will contain at least one of these and should be avoided.

There are a tremendous number of studies showing the harm of these creations such as those listed in "GMO Myths and Legends" available on www.earthopensource.gov. As of this writing, there are sixty-four countries that require labeling or the outright ban of GMOs and GEs. However, the United States does not require labeling on our food products containing ingredients that have been genetically altered, according to www.justlabelit.org. While we don't want to get into a lengthy dissertation of why the United States still allows them, let's just say the other countries have little to lose by banning what they know to be a potentially harmful product while the companies in the United States producing GMOs have much to lose and powerful lobbyists. It is an uphill battle for those of us concerned with GMOs and GEs to get them banned, but more and more consumers are banning together to fight to have labeling. We need to continue to demand the right to have these labeled and hopefully, in time, they will be banished altogether. In the meantime, it's up to you to protect your tummy and your children's tummies from something unrecognizable to the digestive system. Read labels and avoid GMOs and GEs.

Commercial Milk

Ideally, skip milk completely or at least replace standard commercial milk with organic, grass-fed milk. Commercial milk, regardless of whether it's low-fat, 1%, or 2% has too many potential negatives with very few positives. This is especially true for our children since they tend to be the biggest recipients of milk as a health drink. Milk tends to be a mucus-causing drink resulting in inflammation. According to the Physicians Committee for Responsible Medicine's article "What is Lactose Intolerance?" a tremendous number of children and adults are lactose intolerant without knowing it.

Regardless of lactose intolerance, the other point to ponder is what do we get from our commercial milk these days? Some calcium and some added vitamins and minerals. A healthy diet can provide these without the inflammatory qualities of the dairy. In our grandparents' day, milk was loaded with probiotics, vitamins, and enzymes. Today's milk removes the best of these with the heat of pasteurization. In addition, we have crowded feedlots, which create sick cows that produce milk bad for our health. The labeling of "no added synthetic hormones or antibiotics" does not mean it's safe or good. We'll expand on this topic further in our hormones section. I would challenge anyone with health issues to cut out all dairy, including commercial cheese and yogurts, for at least two weeks and see if it makes a difference.

Egg Whites

As a possible source of damage, cut out or reduce egg whites while working on healing the gut. You may or may not have a reaction to eggs, but you will never know unless you cut them out of your diet for a week or two. Many times I hear people are eating healthy by cutting out egg yolk and eating only eggs whites. Unfortunately, this may be the opposite of what our body needs. Egg white contains casein, which can be irritating to the gut while egg yolk has vitally needed cholesterol. I would try cutting out the entire egg and, if your issues ease, add back the yolks to see if your body likes them. Eventually, add the whites if you want, but pay close attention to whether they bother you.

Eggs were another one of those areas I thought didn't matter. I've eaten eggs my entire life. All of my adult life I have also fought with occasional skin breakouts—the painful, under-the-skin kind. Until recently, I could not find a correlation for the breakouts and my daily habits. I had cut out bread and sugar with no results. After considering eggs, I cut them out of my morning breakfast routine, and much to my surprise—and relief—no more breakouts! It never ceases to amaze me how something can be so simple and yet we negate or miss the possibility. What if there is a health issue you or your child is struggling with (eczema, psoriasis, joint pain, tummy pain, etc.), and it's something as simple as eggs (or milk or meat or bread)? Food irritation is our inflammation trigger, so it's worth investigating.

Nightshade Vegetables

Another leaky gut culprit is nightshade veggies. They are called nightshade plants because they prefer shade or the plant flowers at night. Although proteins are the bigger culprits in leaky gut, nightshade veggies, while nutritious, can cause irritation to the gut as well, especially for people with autoimmune conditions. While there are some wonderful antioxidants and nutrition value in these plants, people with autoimmune disorders very well could see a flare up in their condition if they consume the veggies of potatoes, bell peppers, tomatoes, and eggplants. These should be removed from our diets to avoid inflammation and damage while working to heal the gut.

Bad Fats

Another leaky gut factor is bad fats. Avoid hydrogenated and partially hydrogenated oils at all costs. They are in almost every single packaged food on the market including organic foods. When people are concerned with high cholesterol, *these* are the fats they should be dodging. The irony is our medical system tells us to cut out our healthy saturated fats but recommends hydrogenated fats like canola or soybean oils. When I see people baking homemade goodies with a big jug of corn oil or canola oil on the counter, it makes me cringe. To avoid the highly inflammatory qualities of these fats, avoid corn oil, safflower oil, soy oil, and vegetable oil. In addition, many of these are in processed foods so I want to reiterate the importance of reading labels.

If processed oil has been put into packaged foods, it very likely has been heated, bleached, deodorized, or altered in a way that damages the integrity of the fat. Thus, the fat becomes damaged or rancid, which makes it extremely inflammatory and toxic to the body. Even good fats like high-quality sunflower oil become damaged when heated or altered to be used in packaged foods. If a fat has been used in a packaged good, it has more than likely been exposed to high heats and significant damage from the processing. This makes one more reason why we want to avoid packaged foods as much as possible.

Meat

Another major leaky gut culprit is meat. We all assume we need meat protein in our diets. We do need protein, but meat is very difficult to digest. It can greatly spike uric acid levels. Not every meal has to be centered on meat. Our meats today are not the same meats as our ancestors ate. We have crowded feedlots, nitrates, and other additives in the meat. Even if you eat organic, grass-fed meat (the only kind you really should eat), it's still difficult to digest and can still spike uric acid. Limiting meat applies for everyone as far as overall health but especially when working on healing leaky gut. If meat is hard to digest, guess what happens? It sits in the gut, putrefies, and damages the lining. If you do eat meat, don't forget to take your digestive enzymes with HCL to help with digestion.

Gluten

Another damaging factor for leaky gut is gluten. Gluten is far from easy to properly digest. Even if you think you are not gluten intolerant, it is worth cutting it out or greatly reducing it for a week or two to see if some symptoms might be alleviated. You would be surprised what a huge difference this has made for many children and adults. You might think that you'll do many of the things in this book, but you just don't want to go to the effort of eliminating gluten. I get that. It's tough—at least at first—to go without bread and crackers. But, if you struggle with a health issue, it's absolutely vital; it does get easier and easier, and the potential results may be awesome.

I'll admit I was slow to board the gluten-avoidance train. My son was the one to point out that every time Karly ate gluten, she would have severe cramping within an hour. Once he pointed it out, I paid attention. He was right! I became a believer and so did she. Gluten reaction can be powerful in the body. Now remember, her issue was endometriosis—a hormone issue—and yet, the pain and cramping was irritated from her diet. Endo cysts would inflame from the gluten reaction, swell, and cause her severe cramping. Of course, gluten wasn't the only cause of her health problem, but it was a major irritant. What we eat may affect something we think is totally unrelated. Do not discredit the power of gluten intolerance to irritate and inflame.

When you see all the ads or packaging on bread for whole wheat or 12-grain bread as though they are better for you, consider the gluten. For the majority of us today, most grains contain gluten and are an irritant to our digestive system. Therefore, 12 grain or any other whole wheat/grains advertising on standard commercial bread is likely more bad than good for your digestive system. If you eat bread, look for the sprouted grains or ancient grain bread on the market. Ancient grain breads contain natural enzymes (unlike other breads) making them more digestible with less risk of irritation. They are a little heavier than your fluffy white bread, but that's due to the processing of the white bread. Bread was really never meant to be soft and fluffy. You can find ancient grain breads, such as the Ezekiel brand, in the freezer section of most grocery stores. I find it best toasted due to the harder texture of this bread in comparison to soft, white bread.

Be sure to look at the ingredients if you choose to buy gluten-free products. Many of the processed gluten-free products have ingredients that aren't very recognizable to the body or contain our dreaded hydrogenated fats, so it may not be a great replacement for gluten foods. If it says low fat, sugar free, or gluten free, it's a chemical storm. There are likely chemicals, fillers, or synthetics in the food, and that's really no better than gluten.

It may seem as though there is nothing to eat if we cut out gluten since it feels like it's everywhere. There actually are a fair amount of whole foods that do not have gluten such as brown rice, quinoa, and oats. There are breads, pastas, and cereals available at health food stores, online, or the health section of your larger grocery stores made of ancient grains, flax, rice, barley, buckwheat, oats, spelt, quinoa, hemp, or buckwheat. Look for these as it's well worth getting them into your cupboards.

The best way to avoid gluten is to limit or avoid bread, crackers, and pasta while turning your focus on eating your fresh foods as much as possible. After you've been away from these heavier, starchy foods for a few days, you will start to feel lighter, less inflamed and, most importantly, you'll feel better! Pay attention to any and all body reactions that may seem unrelated such as joint pain, sinus problems, ear infections, and diarrhea that flare up after a meal or snack with bread, crackers, grains. Or cut out gluten for at least two weeks and see how you and your child feel (including—and especially—autistic children). You may be like I was with our daughter—greatly surprised!

Eat Healing, Easy-to-digest Foods

Now let's move on to daily things we can do to help that gut of ours. I will caution you to ease into any and all changes or additions to your daily habits. Just because something has potentially good effects for us does not mean we can use them abundantly—at least not at first. Our body needs time to adjust to new foods or drink. It's not always a good idea to think if something is good for me, I'll use more. With *all* foods, supplements, spices, and drinks, we want to always remember moderation. A little of one or even a little of several things is better than loads of one thing. Turmeric is a fabulous healing spice, but too much at one time can irritate. The same applies to ginger or kale. Even liquid aloe vera with all its gentle, healing abilities can cause diarrhea if we use too much at once.

What happens if we bombard the body and get a reaction we don't like? We tend to stop using it when it may be the very protocol or supplement we need. We won't know if we don't give it a good attempt. If you have a reaction (nausea, tired, achy, itchy skin, etc.), discontinue for a few days, then reintroduce at a lesser amount or less often. If you are using small amounts and still getting a reaction you don't like, then you might consider discontinuing. But only if you've given the supplement or food a fair try. Of course, severe reactions could indicate allergy (as opposed to irritant) and you should discontinue. One thing to point out on a reaction to a food is to make sure it's the food and not an additive to the food. I've had people tell me they are allergic to pineapple, for instance. When we discuss the source of the pineapple and we find out it was something like canned pineapple, we have to discuss the can lining chemicals, the added sugar and the ingredients of the syrup over the pineapple. Are you allergic to the pineapple or what's been added to it? The same applies to all food allergies—make sure it's the actual food and not some "extra" that was added to it.

Accordingly, as we discuss these things that can be good for you, remember to ease into their use and pay attention to your body. If your body reacts to a certain spice, supplement, or food, it may be it doesn't like it or it may be too much too fast. One reason I mentioned earlier that your doctor can never help you as much as you help yourself is because he/she can't see your daily reactions to food and environment to know what your body does and does not like. Only *you* can do this.

We rest and ease the burden on our gut with easy-to-digest foods (bone broth, healthy fats), and we offer it healing with supplements like liquid aloe vera, L-Glutamine, apple cider vinegar, etc. We can rest the gut by eating only very light meals of easily digestible foods and liquids for a few days (if no medical issues). Then slowly introduce more foods but, after this, always try to avoid heavy meals and hard-to-digest foods as much as possible.

Organic Greens

Eat organic as much as possible. With all foods, to expend the effort to find organic. The glyphosate sprayed on our produce is powerful at permeating into the plant and our bodies, resulting in extreme damage not only to the gut and hormones but the entire body. We will expand on this topic in our hormones chapter. If you absolutely cannot find or afford organic, soak or spray with a combination of white vinegar and water to try and remove some of the chemicals. Be sure to rinse well with clean water.

93

Most greens are easier to digest and packed with fabulous vitamins and fiber. However, don't forget to chew, chew, chew when it comes to raw greens. Some greens are better slightly blanched or steamed, such as kale or collards as they tend to be some of the greens that can irritate, but many of these greens have their own natural enzymes to help the gut process. Here's the reason, again, most meals began with a salad or soup for hundreds of years. This was to help the stomach start digesting for the rest of the meal of starches and meat that followed.

It's easy to buy a tub of the organic mixed greens, throw a handful on a plate, squeeze fresh lemon, drizzle with olive or hemp oil, and then sprinkle Himalayan or sea salt—*not* processed table salt. This really is delicious and easy. You can even do this with an omelet for breakfast and eat the greens before the omelet. This gets the digestive juices flowing for consuming the eggs, which are much harder to break down and digest. Keep in mind that even though greens can have excellent nutrients, some greens have more than others. Iceberg lettuce—the kind you will most often get at restaurants—is a filler with minimal nutrients. If this is your serving of greens for the day, it's not a good one. (Sorry!) Romaine lettuce, some kale, and arugula (arugula is a strong, bitter green so don't use too much to avoid overwhelming the other greens) are better choices. In addition, using fresh lemon and olive oil (or hemp oil if your heart so desires) is a tremendously better choice than Ranch, blue cheese, western, etc. We do our bodies little good if we choose salad and then pour gunk on top of it. To add insult to injury, most restaurants pour up to ¼ cup of it on the salad. At the very least, ask for the dressing on the side and dip your greens into it. But, better yet, forget it and ask for a couple of lemon wedges and some olive oil.

Bone Broth

Another easy-to-digest food is bone broth. This is one of the best ways to actually help heal our gut lining. Most of the things we list will help avoid damage but don't necessarily heal. Bone broth is healing. What we really want for our gut healing is bone broth, which is a thicker more gelatin version of soup. We get this from the bones of an animal. The purpose is for the MSM, glucosamine, as well as enzymes to literally help heal the gut lining. It's preferable to drink bone broth on an empty stomach so that the lining can absorb it better but drinking it at any time is still helpful. Yes, you can take supplements of glucosamine and MSM, but remember, nothing can ever give us the necessary nutrients and support as well as real food.

Be sure the bones for this broth come from organic, grass-fed animals. A label on the package that claims "no antibiotics or hormones added" is on every meat package you see, and it's *not* the same as organic and grass-fed or pastured animals. You can purchase bone broth online, but again, look for organic and grass-fed or pastured animals. If you purchase it, the broth should have a gelatin-like consistency rather than liquid. Making your own bone broth is much more economical and could even be done in a crockpot. The are many simple recipes for making your own broth online if you Good "bone broth". Our goal here is to get the important nutrients from the inner part of the bones. Dr Axe has a recent new product called Ancient Nutrition Bone Broth Protein which is a powder to make a liquid bone broth. This is a good alternative if you can't find the time to make you own bone broth and you can find it at draxe.com.

Raw Unfiltered Honey

Honey is high in fructose, which isn't a good thing. However, if you're going to use sweeteners, other than Stevia, this would be the one to use. There are many health benefits to raw honey. Raw honey is a unique combination of sugar, minerals, vitamins, trace enzymes, and amino acids. A quality honey has antibacterial, anti-oxidant, and anti-fungal qualities. Choose raw, unfiltered honey for medicinal properties; most honey in grocery stores is highly processed and may even contain additives like corn syrup. Manuka honey comes from the buds on the Manuka bush—a medicinal plant—that gives it even more benefits and can be found in health stores, larger grocery stores or online at Amazon, Thrive Market, and other health sites.

Healthy Fats

I urge you to read more than just my little discussion on this topic or only relying on your doctor's advice. Listen to what he/she has to say, but remember how behind western medicine is on leaky gut. They have the same mindset on healthy (saturated fats) considering them harmful to the body when, actually, the benefits of good fats are well documented. Don't get so concerned about cholesterol or calories that you avoid these without looking into their benefits. Good fats can help burn calories, and that's a good thing! It's vital to have the benefits of saturated fats.

High cholesterol is as related to inflammation as it is to fats. There's no question bad fats, such as vegetable, corn oil, canola, and soybean, are awful for us and surely can contribute to high cholesterol—because they contribute to inflammation—as well as a myriad of other health issues. However, saturated fats, such as coconut oil, butter, and fish oil, can actually soothe the gut to ease inflammation and, as far as calories, these fats listed below can help with our metabolism, aiding us in burning calories. If you want to avoid calories, look toward cutting bread and grains. Don't eliminate your good fats. With that being said, here are some healthy fats that are extremely beneficial to healing leaky gut.

Fish or Krill Oil

I listed these first because they contain omega-3s, which are not in many food sources. Therefore, the majority of us are lacking them. Both fish and krill oil provide omega-3s. The health benefits of omega-3s are through the roof, particularly for brain health. Your gut and your body need fish or krill oil either by eating fish—wild-caught Alaskan salmon is an excellent source (avoid farm-raised)—or through liquid and pill supplementation. While a helpful form of omega-3 can be found in flaxseed, chia, hemp, and a few other foods, the most beneficial form of omega-3—containing both DHA and EPA, which are essential to fighting and preventing both physical and mental disease—can only be found in fish and krill, according to Nature Communications from August 2015.

There are a few differences between krill and fish oil. While fish oil has tremendous advantages, krill oil has many of the same with less risk of being damaged in storage or heat, less risk of toxic Mercury, and less chance of fish burps. There is an abundance of krill on our ocean floor while safe fish oil is short in supply. Thus, the price is much higher on any high-quality fish oil. Be sure to avoid cheap fish oil as the damage from a rancid, poor-quality fish oil will be worse than an insufficiency of fish oil. Again, krill oil may be your safer bet. If you use capsules or liquid and get fish burps, a great way to avoid this is to keep your fish oil capsules in the freezer so they will break down further into the digestive system.

Coconut Oil

It's great to help us digest, fabulous for inflammation, and beneficial for maintaining healthy blood sugar levels. Coconut oil does not provide cholesterol like butter or fish and krill oil, but it has many of its own benefits. Refined coconut oil is my top choice for cooking over all other oils, but organic, *unrefined* coconut oil is better for ingesting raw. I ingest unrefined, organic coconut oil off the spoon several times per day—about a teaspoon each time. But, if this is something you just can't stand, try adding it to oatmeal, green drinks, or your coffee and tea. Some people like to replace the creamer in their coffee (myself included) with coconut oil. This gives it a slightly nutty taste, and makes it a great replacement with positive health benefits rather than the negative from the creamer or milk.

Ghee or Butter

Ghee is butter with the liquid removed; it can be used quite often in place of butter. The cholesterol from both ghee and butter is vital to our systems for hormone function, brain function, joint health, as well as a multitude of cell and nerve interactions. Again, some people like this as an addition to their coffee for the taste as well as the benefits. Buy organic, grass-fed cows' butter, not margarine!

Flax Seed Oil

Flax seed oil contains omega-3s and can support the digestive system to repair and regenerate and digest. It does tend to be easily damaged in the processing so only use high-quality flax oil.

Hemp Oil

This is a great source for omega-3s. You can use it on salads, in green drinks, and straight off the spoon. It does have a stronger taste than coconut oil, but like many things good for you, the taste can be acquired over time.

Olive Oil

Greeks have used large quantities of olive oil for thousands of years. They also have a history of healthy bodies. Drizzle it over your salad or hummus for a healthy perk. Olive oil is great for us but easily damaged in cooking so avoid using it for cooking at high heats.

There are other healthy fats such as grape seed and avocado, but I'm listing the more common ones. If you love to cook, you may want to experiment and read up on some of these other choices.

Spices

We just listed foods (including fats) that soothe. There are a multitude of healing spices that can be beneficial as well. I will caution you, once again, on all spices (or any supplement) to ease into their use and choose high quality sources. Ginger, for example, has been added to food and drink for thousands of years for its soothing benefits but should be started with small amounts at first. I like to blend whole ginger into my green drinks or grate some fresh ginger into a warm cup of water in the mornings or evenings to sip as a tea. Turmeric is another fabulous spice well known for its potential to ease inflammation. As a supplement, turmeric should have black pepper in it to really increase absorption rate. As a whole food or powder, I add it to my green drink. You can add turmeric to many drinks and in your cooking but, once again, small amounts at first and work up. These spices can help with leaky gut by taking stress off the gut lining, which then allows the body's healing process to begin.

Other Gut Helpers

Maintaining proper PH balance is an entire topic-and book-all by itself since it's so vital to our health. This involves alkaline versus acid within the body, especially within our digestive system. Think of alkaline as soothing to the body and too much acid as damaging to the body. One reason green drinks—either blended vegetables (with a little fruit) or juiced vegetables—are so good for us is their nutrients and ability to help us be more alkaline. Although we don't want to be too acidic or too alkaline, we see, by far, more people are acidic than too alkaline. We create acidity in the body from many of the same things that cause gut damage: stress, poor diet, toxins.

Acidic PH can cause the body to be out of balance—losing homeostasis. When that happens, we begin the cycle of imbalance; we invite a host of potential health conditions. Infections and diseases, including osteoporosis and cancer, thrive in an acidic environment. Our body should be at an average pH of 7.36. When you drink a glass of fast food soda or a can of soda, it has a pH of around 2.5. Guess what happens now? All the body systems necessary to try and bring the balance back kick into overdrive. Thus, instead of using its energy to function properly, we are diverting the energy we need for normal day-to-day functions to fight to get that PH balance back. It would take approximately thirty glasses of water just to regain proper PH balance after that soda. Green vegetable juices help restore the body's proper pH; soda disrupts it. The same principle applies to all acidic foods and drink. I'll make a short list of these at the end of the section. The key is to avoid acidity. By alkalizing your body, your cells can heal and regenerate in the manner they are meant to function—including the cells of the digestive lining.

You may see suggestions like adding baking soda in a glass of water, which can be alkaline to the body, but remember moderation is the key. Some people are determined to help the body and go overboard by using a teaspoon of baking soda in their water multiple times throughout the day. This can interfere with enzyme production by making the stomach environment too alkaline; it also could be downright dangerous in large amounts since it may cause stress on the kidneys as well as the entire body. Remember, we should offer small amounts so the body adjusts and adapts slowly. A pinch of baking soda in water a few times per day is all that I personally use; some days I use none to rest my kidneys and let the body work on restoring balance by itself.

Avoid Medications

Another way we can help repair leaky gut is by avoiding chemicals and medications. Medications cause lining damage and lead to inflammation. This includes prescription as well as over-the-counter (OTC) medications. Most people consider OTC medications, such as aspirin, acetaminophen, and ibuprofen, a fairly safe way to deal with pain. It's common to use one of these for a headache, menstrual cramping, leg aches or joint pain. However, they can and will erode the precious gut lining, which once again gives us inflammation and the need to reach for another pain med to start the cycle all over again. Isn't it ironic that those using the "aspirin a day" protocol recommended by their doctors to supposedly help with inflammation are actually contributing to inflammation due to the aspirin irritating and damaging the gut lining?

Support with Supplements

As already mentioned, supplements can be helpful, but nothing will ever provide the vitamins, minerals, and nutrients we need like food. Many people go overboard with supplements taking them by the handfuls several times per day. If we ingest loads of supplements each day, our digestive system and kidneys must process and filter them throughout the day. A healthy digestive system and kidney can hopefully keep up with the filtering but, even if they do, it's hard work on them *and* does what? Puts added stress on them. Therefore, when working on repairing gut lining, some supplements can surely be beneficial, but some is better than too many.

As far as supplements for supporting gut lining repair, by no means is this an all exhaustive list, but these are some supplements that have been shown to offer support to the digestive system so it can repair. They can be found online or any natural health food store. Look for quality, not price. Your health is worth the investment and way too many cheap vitamins and supplements have damaging fillers with little vitamin or nutrient value. Again, I would avoid the big box brands and remember to ease into their use.

Liquid Aloe Vera

This was my go-to supplement when first starting to work on gut health since it has soothing properties to the gut lining. It's affordable, and the one I use is tasteless. It has the potential to support the body's natural processes for maintaining the mucosal lining. I would start with one teaspoon in water twice a day. Some people work up to as much as one ounce per time. The risk is potential diarrhea if you take too much too fast. If that happens, back off on the amount.

You can find this in big gallon jugs (or smaller) in health food stores and online on Amazon and other sites. Since you are going to be ingesting this, it's important to get a good quality brand—be sure its instructions include using it in your water for drinking so that you know it is meant for taking internally. Even if the label on the jug says it's for internal use, flip the jug over to read the ingredients. I have seen some that say drinkable but then show a list of words I can't pronounce. Most of them are preservatives. Be sure the label only says aloe vera and perhaps water. That should be it. I will list some sources for liquid aloe vera at the end of this chapter. Liquid aloe vera can be good for our pet as well. My dog gets this every day although I put it in his food instead of water so he's sure to take it.

L-Glutamine

This is a supplement that usually comes in either capsule or powdered form. It is the preferred food of the cells of the small intestine to support and nourish the digestive system. Thus, it works somewhat like a Band-Aid to the lining while you work on healing.

Quercetin

This is another one that can help restore normal gut-lining tissue. Quercetin supports a healthy gut by sealing the gut and helping the gut seal the lining. Quercetin also reduces the release of histamine, which is common in food intolerance or sensitivities.

DGL/ 4 Licorice Root

This is a supplement that normally comes in a chewable tablet or powder form. It may help balance and improve enzymes production in the stomach as well as support maintenance of the mucosal lining.

Zinc

Zinc is required for growth and healing—particularly important to cells that have a rapid turnover rate such as the cells in the small intestine.

Fish and Krill Oil

Here are fish and krill oil again! Hopefully, it's coming through loud and clear that fish or krill oil should be part of every person's daily regimen. The omega-3s in both of these are difficult to source for most of us. Fish was once a regular meal in most homes, but that is no longer the case due to rushed lifestyles plus the difficulty of purchasing fish without some contamination. Fish and krill oil support proper nutrient absorption, have anti-inflammatory properties, and provide badly needed omega-3s to help the body with repair. However, be sure to get high-quality fish oil or the additives and oxidation will outweigh any benefit received. As aforementioned, krill oil is less susceptible to oxidation and easier sourcing so it's a good replacement for fish oil.

Broad Spectrum Daily Vitamin

While food is our primary way to get nutrients, it's hard to get all our nutrients from our food due to depleted soil nutrient levels, processed foods, and of course, a less than optimal digestive system. Therefore, a whole food multivitamin is a good idea. Once again, be sure to look for a high-quality, whole food vitamin to avoid damaging fillers. Vitamins can be irritating to an empty stomach, which would more than defeat our purpose of wanting to help the body so be sure to use them with food.

So, there we have it. Habits, foods, changes, and supplements we can use to help repair leaky gut. Once again, *why* do we want to work on leaky gut? Here a few reasons:

- Damaging foods and habits erode the lining of our digestive system.
- A damaged lining allows toxins and invaders outside the digestive system into the bloodstream.
- These toxins do not belong in the bloodstream and are highly inflammatory.
- Inflamed glands, joints, muscles, etc. *will* cause pain and disruption of their normal function.

When we soothe any inflamed body part, we can feel tremendously better—not just in the area of inflammation but throughout the body. A leaky gut is a compromised, damaged, inflamed part of the body. Remember the approximate area of the digestive system? One full tennis court. Take the lining for that entire system and imagine it inflamed. How could this *not* make a difference in our health? How could it not affect every single body system in the human body?

If we ease the stress and damage on that susceptible, mucosal lining, we allow it to begin the healing process. We support it to help it repair itself thereby easing the stress on the entire body. Good things happen in the body and brain with less stress on the digestive system with the end result of less inflammation! You might very possibly improve your health issues, including autoimmune conditions, by improving the health of your gut lining.

I list suggestions for support below but do not get overwhelmed. Remember to only pick a few to start and then go from there. I have also listed a beginner's list of only a few things for supporting the entire digestive system at the end of the gut health discussion. Start with that list and add from the list at the end of each section on the Focus Four as you develop good additions and habits from the beginner's list.

Sum It Up

In order to repair our gut lining, the second step in the Focus Four, we must properly support the digestive lining. Here are the necessary steps to heal leaky gut:

- Avoid and/or reduce stress.
- Avoid heavy meals and damaging foods.
- Eat healing, easy-to-digest foods.
- Avoid chemicals and medications.
- Support with supplements.

Cheat Sheet to Repairing Gut Lining

Healing Foods   -NOT-   Damaging Foods

- Bone Broth
- Steamed Veggies
- Light Meals
- Health Fats

- Milk
- Gluten
- Egg Whites (Casein)
- Bad Fats (Margarine, Canola)

Easy-to-Digest Foods   -NOT-   Hard-to-Digest Foods

- Oatmeal
- Ancient Grains Bread
- Basmati Rice
- Quinoa
- Nuts and Seeds
- Yogurt (unpasteurized/plain)

- Microwave Popcorn
- Large, Heavy Meals
- Meat
- Bread
- Potatoes

Alkaline Foods and Drinks   -NOT-   Acidic Foods and Drinks

- Green Tea
- Cucumbers
- Beets
- Baking Soda
- Lemon
- Apple Cider Vinegar

- Coffee
- Alcohol
- Carbonated Water
- Soda (Diet & Regular)

Healthy Fats (Organic Only)	-NOT-	Fats to Avoid
• Fish and Krill Oil		• Margarine
• Unrefined Coconut Oil		• Canola Oil
• Flax Oil		• Soybean Oil
• Hemp Oil		• Vegetable Oil
• Butter and Ghee		• Corn Oil
• Sunflower Oil		

Healthy Supplements and Spices	-NOT-	Damaging Supplements and Spices
• L-Glutamine		• Cheap supplements and fillers
• Liquid Aloe Vera		• Aspirin
• Ginger		• Acetaminophen
• Turmeric		• Ibuprofen
• Quercetin		
• Zinc		

Chapter Seven: Restore Bacteria and Microbiome Balance

We've now covered the first and second steps of the Focus Four. As a reminder of our goal, let's review our list:

1. Recharge Digestion: break down our food and get our nutrients
2. Repair Gut Lining: heal and maintain the digestive system lining and keep toxins out of bloodstream to help avoid inflammation
3. Restore Bacteria and Microbiome Balance: support our immunity and nervous system health
4. Rid Toxins and Elimination: poop to get those toxins out of the body

Just like the first two items on the list, the third is very important. If your doctor told you about a prescription for that little pill I mentioned earlier that would help with up to 80 percent of your immune system, wouldn't there be a line out the door for this pill? If it were a prescription medication, the media would be highlighting its miraculous abilities. And yet, it's unlikely you hear about it at a health appointment for you or your child. The good news is you possess that little pill through the knowledge of supporting your microbiome balance.

This chapter discusses ways to support your immune system. With so much potential to impact our immune system, there's no question this information is important, and potentially life-changing. If you have been reading awhile and your brain is tired, take a break. Come back when you are fresh because this topic is literally a game changer for your health. The best part is this game changer isn't a procedure or an injection. It involves no prescriptions or doctor visits. You don't need a specialist or a surgeon. It simply involves something you and you alone can support. It's within your control, and it's actually quite easy.

Balance

So, what is this amazing thing? It's replenishing and bringing balance to the microbiome/bacteria of our digestive system through either a capsule that delivers its contents of multiple strains of bacteria or through fermented foods that also provide many strains. With this help to provide gut microbiome balance, we have a powerful ability to resist infection, bacteria, viruses, and invaders. Without this equilibrium, our body is very susceptible to these invaders. In our bodies, we *must have* a proper bacteria and microbiome balance to support a healthy immune system, brain communication, skin health, and literally every function in the body. Why should we be concerned with our bacteria and microbiome balance? Here are a few reasons:

- Microbiome and bacteria balance is key to up to 80 percent of immunity, according to Dr. Mercola (www.mercola.com).

- Neuron receptors in our microbiome and bacteria in our gut communicate with the brain; if one is upset or inflamed, so is the other.

- Microbiome imbalance reflects in our skin through conditions such as eczema or psoriasis or a variety of other skin issues.

- According to the 2011 article "Role of Gut Microbiota in Defining Human Health" (**www.ncbi.com**), there are a multitude of major health conditions and diseases linked to microbiome imbalance including candida, rheumatoid arthritis, diabetes, IBS, and more.

- The balance of microbiome can influence behavior and brain health shown by studies that have found autistic children differ in their microbiome compared to healthy children. In particular, it was shown they tend toward having fewer beneficial bacteria, such as Bifidobacterium, as cited in the 2013 abstract "Fecal Microbiota and Metabolome of Children with Autism and Pervasive Developmental Disorder Not Otherwise Specified" (www.journals.plos.org).

While leaky gut, the subject of the last chapter, involves holes in the digestive lining, microbiome and bacteria balance involves supporting healthy bacteria within that digestive lining. Many people think of bacteria as a bad thing, but for overall health, nothing could be further from the truth. What is problematic and the cause of rising health issues is an imbalance of the bad bacteria to the good bacteria. We actually want and need some of both. These microbiome and bacteria are teeming throughout the inside of your body, but they are also teeming on the outside of the body (the skin). These are *living* organisms that communicate with each other. When all is well, they communicate in a positive way to help your body function properly. When they are disrupted or imbalanced, their communication is also interrupted. This is where the core of many health conditions begins.

If you grasp the importance of microbiome balance, you will hopefully incorporate habits into your daily life to maintain a healthy balance. This has potential for major impact on your or your children's health—with hopes if you are wanting to avoid such things as ear and sinus infections, for instance, you will be diligent on supporting their microbiome and bacteria balance with probiotics and fermented foods. These are important not only for current health conditions but also for long-term health.

The Connection

There are literally trillions of bacteria and microbiome in and on our bodies. This applies to our children, our parents, grandparents, and ourselves. It applies to every single human being. We have more bacteria (good and bad) than human cells. Therefore, if the core makeup of our entire body is not in balance, we are subject to a host of ailments. I call this the dance of the bacteria because if the gut environment isn't functioning properly, there is an imbalance in not only your gut but ultimately throughout the rest of your body. This statement is the very essence of your being. Bad microbiome flourishing in your digestive system create a disruption in the *entire* body—not only in the digestive system.

There is a symbiotic relationship between the gut bacteria and your immune system (colds, flu, ear and sinus infection), your ability to handle stress, your mood (anxiety, panic attacks) as well as your skin (eczema, acne, psoriasis) and many other conditions in the body—all due to this important balance.

Your skin is the "canary in the coal mine" for overall health. Although it's rare to have a doctor discuss bacteria balance in your digestive system if you have skin issues, they really should consider it. Dr. Mercola's 2011 article "Probiotics Send Signals From Your Gut to Your Skin" claims you have up to one million bacteria living on every square inch of your skin (www.mercola.com). They exist even after you wash your face. Hearty little guys, aren't they? These microbiomes on the skin are greatly influenced by what we eat since, ultimately, what we eat will reflect on our skin; what goes in reflects without.

It's also rare for your doctor to say the possibility for anxiety, panic attacks, or the inability to handle stress could be related to a microbiome balance. If the gut and brain communicate (and they do!), our brain health *will* be disrupted when the gut microbiome is imbalanced. As Peter Andrey Smith wrote in the June 2015 *New York Times* article "Can the Bacteria in Your Gut Affect Your Mood?":

> Anxiety, depression and several pediatric disorders, including autism and hyperactivity, have been linked with gastrointestinal abnormalities.... [L]ast September, the National Institute of Mental Health awarded four grants worth up to $1 million each to spur new research on the gut microbiome's role in mental disorders, affirming the legitimacy of a field that had long struggled to attract serious scientific credibility.... It seems plausible, if not yet proved, that we might one day use microbes to diagnose neurodevelopmental disorders, treat mental illnesses and perhaps even fix them.

Although the above article states it's not yet proven, it may be a little behind since a study just released (May 6, 2016) backs the effect of balanced microbiome and using supplemental support through probiotics as beneficial to mental health. According to the abstract from Yakult Central Institute, "A novel clinical trial was conducted in healthy medical students under examination stress conditions. It was demonstrated that the daily consumption of lactic acid bacteria gave health benefits to prevent the onset of stress-associated abdominal symptoms together with a good change of gut-microbiota in healthy medical students" (www.http://www.ncbi.nlm.nih.gov/). As I visit with attendees at speaking engagements and my wellness consultations, I far too often hear of someone struggling with mental health conditions such as anxiety or depression and yet gut health has not been presented to them as a possible contributor. Instead, they are given brain-numbing medications that ironically disrupt gut health even more. Although I would never interfere with a person's medical prescription, what I would encourage is a high amount (easing into it) of probiotics with a variety of strains as well as fermented foods to see if they might help with the communication between brain and gut.

The same applies to conditions like IBS, Crohn's, and colitis. They can likely be eased if not greatly improved by working on microbiome balance. Western medicine's answers are antibiotics (the opposite, in the long run to microbiome support), steroids, and pain meds. When we have to race to the bathroom, it's the body saying it doesn't like what's going in your intestines and digestive system. Inflammation and disruption of microbiome lead to chaos whereas a calm and soothing system leads to healing. The impact of gut health resonates throughout our body. You may be able to help health issues that, up to now, weren't improving! You can now take positive steps—by yourself—and very possibly without a multitude of invasive tests and specialists.

Now let's discuss some ways you can support and restore the balance in your digestive system and, ultimately, contribute to better balance of all your body systems.

Probiotics

I've mentioned this before but will say it again. If I took only one supplement, vitamin, oil, or treatment, it would be a high-quality probiotic.

This is prime support for our immune system! Probiotics, along with your fermented foods, are the best way to maintain and regain balance in the digestive system. Supplementing with probiotics and eating fermented foods should be not only a daily habit for a health condition but an ongoing habit for the rest of your life to help prevent health conditions.

Let's take a look at what probiotics and fermented foods are as well why we want them. Think of probiotics as food for your immune system. They actually *are* food for your bacteria balance. The best probiotic capsule on the market will normally provide *billions* of good bacteria. You will see them on store shelves with anywhere from 3 to 150 billion. Personally, I don't consider three billion enough for the average adult but perhaps to introduce them to your system or for children they would be helpful. An average adult might use one that provides 10 to 50 billion. Using too much too soon might possibly cause diarrhea so ease into the higher amounts. If you are someone who struggles with diarrhea issues, you should eventually see some help in reducing, if not eliminating it by supplementing with probiotics. In many cases, diarrhea is a *symptom* of severe bacteria imbalance and probiotics might just be your new best friend.

You shouldn't see or feel any harmful side effects with probiotics as you introduce them to your system other than the possible aforementioned diarrhea or short term "die off" symptoms we will discuss in the upcoming paragraph on this subject. Often, people tend to not take *enough* capsules and/or using one with a low amount of bacteria count (like three billion bacteria) for long-term use. When they don't see a difference in their health, they may decide there's no validity to this whole probiotic idea and stop using them. As you use the probiotics, see how you react. In most areas, you may have a flurry of activity before it eventually settles down. Does your skin clear? Does your diarrhea settle down? If not, use more capsules after you take the time to ease into them. If yes, continue what you are doing.

Probiotic supplements are a tad pricey for the average person to add to the budget. Remember, if you see one that costs much less than most brands, they most likely are also cheap quality. It's a careful, extensive process to obtain microbiome and bacteria, put them in capsules, and deliver them to market without destroying the delicate balance of those little fellas. However, if you want to look and feel healthy, it's a good investment to spend your money on probiotics (even before makeup and clothes). The interior reflects the exterior. The interior will never be in balance without bacteria and microbiome support. Use your high-quality probiotics!

Like many supplements, there is an array of probiotic capsules on the market, which can overwhelm us. Don't get hung up on prebiotics versus probiotics or trying to learn all the different strains of bacteria. If you have a health condition and want to research whether you need a higher amount of one strain, that's something you may consider. But the average person is well served by a probiotic capsule that contains a variety of strains, which are what you should find in most of your high-quality brands (I will mention a few at the end of this section). Most likely the highest quality probiotic supplements are going to be in a refrigerated area to help prevent destroying the bacteria in the capsules. You likely won't find the high-quality probiotics with a drugstore or big box store label (Walgreens, CVS, Target, Wal-Mart). I wouldn't suggest using the store label brands because they don't specialize in this area, but these stores might possibly carry decent brands such as ReNew Life, Pure, Natures Garden, or Nature's Bounty. If you purchase online, I like Dr. Mercola (www.mercola.com) or Dr. Axe (www.draxe.com) in addition to those just listed. There are many other good brands; these are just a few I like. Research to see what brand fits your needs and price range. The key is to look for one from a company that specializes in supplements.

One final thought is that the microbiome found in our soil are the most powerful of all probiotic strains. A little dirt on the carrot from the garden isn't a bad thing as long as your garden isn't sprayed with chemicals; it might be a great idea to leave a little on the garden foods instead of scrubbing them squeaky clean. I would, however, scrub the garden foods from the supermarket to make sure there are no chemicals, waxes, or bacteria.

Fermented Foods

The other side of the coin for microbiome and bacteria balance is to consume fermented foods. The best probiotic in the world provides billions of needed bacteria while fermented food can provide *trillions*. This is why we want to add fermented foods as much or more than probiotic supplements. It's also one reason (amongst many) why our grandparents had less gut and health issues than our generation. However, fermented foods versus probiotic supplements provide different strains of bacteria, so it's good to vary what you use and, ideally include *both* probiotic supplements as well as the fermented foods to support and balance the bacteria in the body.

What are fermented foods? These are foods our grandparents consumed daily like unpasteurized yogurt, sauerkraut, pickles, or home-canned pickled vegetables. However, in our grandparents' day, these things were made at home likely using only chemical free ingredients with no unhealthy additives. The problem we have today is that our foods are pasteurized. Once undergoing the process of heating the food/liquid for pasteurization, we have damaged the bacteria in the food and have a huge drop in the population of natural bacteria and microbiome population in that food. Therefore, when a famous actress promotes her yogurt because it has good pre/probiotics, it's at least a good way to make people aware we need them. As long as the product she promotes has been pasteurized, however, the benefit is small compared to an unpasteurized version. Add to the fact that most yogurts on the shelves have preservatives, sugar, dyes, and more. Overall, it's better than cookies but not maybe not nearly as healthy as we are led to believe. Yes, there is a slight risk of illness from unpasteurized foods, but there's a bigger risk, over a lifetime of reduced microbiome/bacteria in our foods, of health issues from an imbalanced population in the gut.

What's a person to do to get our badly needed bacteria and microbiome? Look for some of the following foods that are unpasteurized or minimally pasteurized. If you can find them, you will want to be sure they ideally from a clean farm where cows (or goats) are free to eat in pastures that have not been chemically sprayed. (This is getting to be a difficult request these days.)

- Yogurt: As discussed, it would be ideal to get unpasteurized, but that is difficult to find. At the very least, get organic (ideally) and plain flavored. Add your own flavor rather than the artificial flavor added by many of the commercial brands; they are usually laden with extras you are trying to avoid. Add berries, cinnamon, or a drop of vanilla, but choose the plain-flavored yogurt over flavored. Yogurt does have lactose, which can make it harder on the digestive system. My preference would be kefir.

- Kefir: This is similar to yogurt, but the kefir grains help digest the lactose that is difficult to digest. Remember we are trying to get foods that are easy-not difficult-to digest so kefir is a good choice. You can find kefir on many store shelves in the dairy section. The same applies to kefir as yogurt; avoid the flavored kind and add your own healthier options. Since it is a tad thinner than yogurt, I add a good quality vanilla flavored protein mix to it along with berries. The protein mix thickens it up just a tad, making it more like yogurt.

- Sauerkraut: I know it smells, but try to look at it like pickles; it's a bit tart and adds flavor. Many times, I put it on the side of my plate when I have a salad. Once you get used to this, it's good!

- Kimchi: This is sauerkraut with veggies and a few peppers. I prefer this to plain sauerkraut, as I like the bite in it. Again, add it to the side of salads and consume with your salad if you don't like it by itself.

- Kombucha: This is a fermented drink that comes in a variety of flavors. It's actually a little fizzy like soda so if you are trying to make the transition from soda to health drinks, give kombucha a try. Be sure to read the label on the bottle to make sure there are no added sugars or preservatives. Kombucha can bother some people's gut lining so I might hold off on this one until you've done some healing to the gut lining or try smaller amounts to start.

There are other fermented food choices but these are the most common and therefore easiest to find. When you begin adding good bacteria to your diet through probiotics and fermented foods, it's possible you experience what's known as die-off symptoms. You might (or might not) experience dizziness, headaches, low fever, skin rash, upset tummy, and a general flu-like feeling. These are all natural parts of die-off symptoms known as a detoxification reaction labeled the Herxheimer Reaction. This is one reason we say a person may feel worse before they feel better when first venturing into natural health alternatives. It's also why we recommend easing into any new food or liquid when first introducing them to the body. While it might be uncomfortable, it is not dangerous but a good reason to ease into use. You might slightly decrease the number of fermented foods or probiotics (but don't quit) and also drink loads of water to help the body catch up on the elimination process. The bacteria's die-off symptoms shouldn't last long and, on the upside, you should be feeling better soon. So continue with your fermented foods and probiotics. It's well worth it!

More Balance Helpers

We just covered what I consider the first place to begin supporting microbiome balance—probiotics and fermented foods. Start with these and then move on to a few additional things that help us maintain this balance.

Digestive Enzymes

Remember these from our digestion section? Not only are digestive enzymes important to digest your food for nutrients but also so we get the food out of the stomach. If your food sits in the stomach too long, the body sends in extra enzymes which upsets balance plus the large particles of undigested food make for a great meal for the unfriendly bacteria we are trying to avoid. Therefore, undigested food from inadequate digestive enzymes can ultimately disrupt the microbiome balance of the digestive system.

Stress

Again and again, we will see stress as the problem child in our body systems.

ESSENTIAL GUT & HORMONE WELLNESS

The effects of chronic stress disrupt the bacteria and microbiome balance, plus—as discussed earlier—it erodes the gut lining, contributing to leaky gut. This upsets our PH balance and improper production of our enzymes for digestion. Remember our earlier discussion? All the supplements and healthy foods in the world can't solve our issues if we continue to introduce high stress in our daily lives. Our upcoming chapter on stress better details its effect on our lives and ways to work on stress reduction to calm ourselves.

Repair Leaky Gut

We have this vicious cycle between bacteria imbalance causing leaky gut and vice versa. Leaky gut affects bacteria balance, and imbalanced bacteria impacts leaky gut. This proves, once again, that the body is an intrinsic machine. Support to proper microbiome and bacteria balance becomes as high a priority as healing leaky gut because both functions literally depend on the other. If we have a damaged gut lining, we lose the effectiveness of the soldiers guarding the castle, which ultimately affects our microbiome balance as the bad guys get out of control. This is just one reason we work on leaky gut (the second action of the Focus Four) in conjunction with supporting our microbiome and bacteria balance.

Fiber

Soluble fiber found in oatmeal, beans, apples, sprouted seeds, and blueberries is great for supporting the balance of microbiome. Fiber is important for many different things in terms of your digestion. Actually, when we consume fiber, we often consume too much insoluble fiber and not enough soluble fiber. Insoluble fiber found in whole wheat bread, nuts, and brown rice is more abundant in today's diet while soluble fiber, also known

121

as prebiotics, is really what supports the growth of good bacteria in the gut.

Avoid Antibiotics

If you must take antibiotics, it's vital to double or triple your probiotics and fermented foods after antibiotic treatment. It's encouraging to know more pharmacists are now informing people to use probiotics when they pick up their antibiotic prescription; this means western medicine is beginning to acknowledge the benefits of probiotics. Antibiotics can cause major disruption in the microbiome balance that very likely will *not* rebalance without intervention from you in the way of probiotics and fermented foods. If you don't offer a significant amount of probiotics to rebalance, you may be back on another prescription before long. This also applies to our children.

A common problem is when we feel like we just can't get our children or ourselves off the merry-go-round of sick-antibiotics-sick-antibiotics. This normally begins when we catch a bug that's going around, so we take antibiotics. We recover for a few days or weeks and then we (or our children) are sick again with the ultimate result being *more* antibiotics. Why does this keep happening? One reason is the bacteria balance was never reestablished after the first round of antibiotics, leaving us susceptible to the next bad bug (remember—up to 80% of immunity) circulating at school, work, or daycare. Increasing probiotics and fermented foods after antibiotic use is a great way to rebuild balance and immunity so your immune system can hopefully have good resistance to the next bug that comes around.

Avoid Birth Control Pills

Approximately 80 percent of sexually active women in the United States have used birth control pills, according to www.guttmacher.org. Like antibiotics, oral contraceptives can be a big enemy to the balance of bacteria in the gut due to interference with optimal trace elements (magnesium, zinc, selenium, and phosphorous) absorption and disruption of normal hormone interactions as only a partial list of side effects of the contraceptive pill says the 2011 abstract from Cape Peninsula University of Technology's Department of Biomedical Sciences (**http://www.ncbi.nlm.nih.gov/**).

Since such a high number of women have used birth control likely causing disrupted bacteria and microbiome balance and since there is a tie between gut microbiome balance and brain activity, this might be a reason why a 2007 study from Alfred Psychiatry Research Centre shows depression as a side effect of the pill. However, a study mentioned in the Morbidity and Mortality Weekly Report entitled "Antidepressant Prescription Claims Among Reproductive-Aged Women with Private Employer-Sponsored Insurance, United States 2008-2013" shows we are seeing a 15.4 percent rate of younger women using anti-depressant medications. It frustrates me to think of the number of years Karly suffered with depression while also on birth control pills prescribed in an attempt to manage her Endo symptoms. Unfortunately, we didn't make the connection. It makes you wonder if things could have been different. Obviously, not in her case but perhaps in yours if you are on birth control pills, are struggling with depression and have never heard of the birth control connection. If you are on a contraceptive pill and if you also struggle with emotional health issues, I would encourage you to consider getting off the pill to help balance microbiome of your gut and hopefully ease brain health interference.

Avoid Chemicals

Foods and chemicals can disrupt and alter gut bacteria. This includes antibacterial hand soaps found everywhere. It also includes foods such as your packaged and processed foods, artificial sweeteners, sodas (especially diet soda), sugar, and fructose. The other big culprit is the chemical glyphosate found in most non-organic foods. Glyphosate popularity rose tremendously with the introduction of GMO foods that allow the plant to withstand higher levels of chemicals without killing the plant. By no means does that make it safe for us.

Avoid City Chlorinated Water

While chlorine is great for your pool and also keeps your city out of lawsuits by killing bacteria for safe drinking water, it also can disrupt or kill valuable bacteria in your gut. Most water pitchers with filters will remove chlorine (although they don't remove fluoride). If you purchase a water pitcher with a filter, be sure to read and make sure it removes chlorine.

Avoid Sugar

Bad bacteria feed on sugar—it's one reason our body craves sugar. Hopefully, you have heard of candida, and that it's not a good bacteria. When we have a diet high in sugar (which is typical), candida and other bad bacteria multiply, embed, invade, and overwhelm our good bacteria to make for a very disrupted microbiome balance.

Sugar comes in very many forms such as cane sugar, syrup, fructose, sucrose, etc. If your food comes in a box or bag, sugar will almost always be listed as one of the ingredients. Read your labels and learn to spot the hidden sugar. Remember pasta, potatoes, and other starches turn to sugar in the body.

Avoid Packaged Foods

Too often a person trying to work on better health swaps out cookies for low-fat or gluten-free cookies. I'll remind you if *any* package, regardless whether it's cookies, crackers, or cereal says, "sugar free" or "low fat" or "gluten free," think chemical storm because that's exactly what it is. Read the package; see if you can find even one recognizable or healthy ingredient. Packaged foods are one of the big flaws in the American diet. That's the best way to think of them. Look at a box of mac & cheese or dinner in a box to use with chicken, hamburger, or tuna. We already know the starch-based part of it (macaroni or rice) is not healthy. The remaining portion of the box is the powdered mix, which is anything but beneficial for our body. Once again, read the ingredients. See how many healthy ingredients there really are; I'm betting almost zero. The best way to get any type of chemically free food is by eating whole food.

Maintain Proper PH Balance

Just like with leaky gut, we also want to watch our acidic versus alkaline balance. If we have an acidic environment in the body, this contributes to microbiome imbalance. Our PH balance—acid versus alkaline—is a key component to proper microbiome balance. How do we maintain proper PH balance? Many of the same foods and principles as we discussed for leaky gut and digestion are the same principles for avoiding acidity. Squeeze lemon in water; add apple cider vinegar to water; eat greens; avoid damaging foods such as gluten, sugar, and dairy. Avoid excessive caffeine and alcohol. There are more PH-supporting habits and foods, but the aforementioned give you a good start.

Momma's Gut and Pregnancy

I feel it's important to discuss this subject before completing our microbiome balance section. If you want to help your child get off to a good start in life, it's vital those planning to get pregnant be aware that microbiome and bacteria balance is inherited from mama to baby. We are seeing skyrocketing statistics on children with issues like allergies, eczema, asthma, ear infections, pneumonia as mentioned in the 2011 Journal Issue: Children with Disabilities, volume 22 (www.futureofchildren.org). One study mentioned in the 2010 article "Prevalence of Chronic Illness in US Kids Has Increased" (www.medscape.com) shows the rate of chronic health conditions among children in the United States increased from 12.8 percent in 1994 to 26.6 percent in 2006.

Why are they such a problem today? Let's consider that so many young women are struggling with poor microbiome and bacteria balance due to birth control pills, high-sugar diet, and stress. Since our doctors do not discuss any of these as part of their health care regiment, most of these women have no idea they have a poor balance. Now these same young ladies have babies who would normally get healthy microbiomes as they pass through the birth canal. The problem is if the mother doesn't have good balance, how can she share it with her baby? Thus, baby is born without the protection of good bacteria and microbiome balance. There are studies mentioned in the February 2011 issue of *Canadian Medical Association Journal* showing babies born via C-section have even fewer beneficial bacteria and are at higher risk for various health problems. These babies get even less of the good bacteria and microbiome balance, so it's even more important to get probiotic support.

Hopefully, the baby looks all pink, darling, and healthy. This is due to the fact the mother's body, while pregnant, was giving baby the best of what she had. However, once baby is born, they begin getting exposed to the toxins and bacteria and viruses of our world. It's normal that they get exposed. What is not normal is baby's potentially poor microbiome and bacteria balance, which can lead to poor immunity and protection. The toxins in our environment, such as fabric softeners, air fresheners, cleaning products, hairspray, perfume, and the herbicides on most fruits and veggies, considered safe is also abnormal. Even infant formulas contain as much as 50 percent sugar, which wreaks havoc on an already weak immune system. Add the increased vaccine schedule that has skyrocketed from *seven* when I was a child to thirty-six vaccines prior to entering school, according to "History of Vaccine Schedule" on www.vactruth.com. Children today are bombarded with a multitude of factors causing disruption to their microbiome balance. To make matters worse, when these susceptible babies get sick, they receive antibiotics, which literally devastates bacteria balance even more (and sets them up for another round of illness in the near future).

We won't get into vaccinating versus not vaccinating in this discussion, but we do at least need to recognize that a weakened immune system cannot possibly handle the attack on the body that multiple vaccines in one visit present. Most, if not all, of the childhood illnesses we see today are listed as a side effect on the vaccine inserts. Many parents assume the vaccinations do no harm because the child doesn't get the illness from which the vaccine is intended to protect. However, parents are not made aware that a compromised immune system sets baby up for a slew of other potential childhood illnesses from the attack on the immune system as a result of the vaccine. Protect baby by building their gut bacteria immunity and removing the toxins in their world prior to vaccinations should you choose to vaccinate.

Ladies, it's super important to take care of your gut health not only for you but also for your little one. Don't wait until you are pregnant to start focusing on this area; it's a process that can take some time and you don't want to wait until pregnancy to pay attention to it. If you know you are having a C-section, research seeding. This is where the mother swipes a gauze pad vaginally and puts it in a sealed container to use inside baby's mouth after birth in an attempt to help transfer some of mama's microbiomes to baby.

Once baby is born, probiotics can and should be introduced to help support and rebuild their bacteria balance. Open the capsule and add it to their bottle if baby is bottle-fed. Open the capsule and apply the powder around the nipples if you are breastfeeding or swipe the contents inside the mouth. If baby gets formula, study and read on the different brands of formula and watch out for the sugar. Nothing could be worse for baby's start in life than to give them sugar. This applies to infancy and throughout childhood. As the child gets foods introduced, try adding some kefir to their diets for good microbiome-support boost.

As we review this chapter, you will see a repeat of many of the items helpful for proper microbiome balance are some of those we listed for proper digestion and leaky gut. The beauty of this means we aren't learning a multitude of new foods, supplements, and protocols with each section we discuss on gut health. Incorporating those in the upcoming list means you are supporting more than one of the Focus Four in the digestive function list. This emphasizes that we don't need complicated protocols. Offer the basics and let the gut—and body—do the rest.

Remember, this isn't about what foods *you* like; it's about what your *body* will like (and need). So even if it's not your favorite food, start incorporating small amounts to get used to it if you really do want to improve gut health and teach your little ones the foundation of good health.

Sum It Up

Once again, why would we want to be concerned with our bacteria and microbiome balance?

- Microbiome and bacteria balance are the foundation to body immunity.
- Neuron receptors in our microbiome and bacteria in our gut communicate with the brain; good brain health is vitally linked to gut health.
- Microbiome imbalance reflects on the skin.
- There are forty major health conditions and diseases linked to microbiome imbalance including depression, arthritis, IBS, and cancer.

Support healthy microbiome and bacteria balance in the digestive system. You can do this by:

- o Avoiding stress
- o Consuming fermented foods
- o Supporting with probiotics and supplements
- o Eating alkaline versus acid foods for healthy PH balance
- o Avoiding antibiotics, medications, and chemicals

Cheat Sheet for Restoring Bacteria and Microbiome Balance

Fermented Foods (Unpasteurized)   -NOT-   Pasteurized Foods

• Kimchi

• Kefir (Plain)

• Yogurt (Plain)

• Kombucha

• Sauerkraut, Pickles, Green Olives

• Pasteurized, Flavored Yogurts

• Pasteurized Kefir

Good Environment   -NOT-   Disruptive Environment

• Filtered Spring Water

• Organic, Chemical-Free Foods

• Unfiltered, Chlorinated City Water

• Non-Organic Foods

• Foods exposed to Glyphosate

• Sugar

Alkaline Foods and Drinks   -NOT-   Acidic Foods and Drinks

• Green Tea

• Celery

• Cucumbers

• Beets

• Coffee

• Alcohol

• Soda (Diet and Regular)

• Carbonated Water

• Chlorinated City Water

Supplements	-NOT-	Medications

Supplements

- Probiotics
- Digestive Enzymes

-NOT-

Medications

- Antibiotics
- Birth Control Pills

Chapter Eight: Rid Toxins and Elimination

We've covered the first three steps of the Focus Four. Last but not least is the topic of elimination—something we (hopefully) do on a daily basis. We may even think it's a simple topic and might want to skip over this section. This section is brief but a big part of digestive health, and there are always more tidbits to learn.

Eliminate to Eliminate

Think about the word elimination. We eliminate, get rid of, remove. That's exactly what we want to do when we visit the bathroom. We want to excrete the toxins that our digestive system, in its amazing ability, has put a tremendous amount of energy into filtering, sorting, and directing to the colon.

Children and teenagers love poop jokes, but by the time we are adults, we start to realize elimination is no laughing matter. We all eliminate. It's our main body function designed to rid toxins—germs, bacteria, solid material—from the body. However, if we don't go on a regular basis, we don't eliminate the toxins from our body. So where do these toxins go? They don't just disappear...

Once again, I want you to think how your poop smells. Imagine these smelly, disgusting toxins as living organisms that *should* have been eliminated. Now imagine them taking advantage that the body didn't get rid of them as scheduled. They are crazy happy about this because their very existence, which had been threatened by the process of elimination, has just been given a second chance. They get to reabsorb into your colon lining and, if you have damaged gut lining, eventually into your bloodstream to live, thrive, and multiply. This is a great deal for the toxins (live bacteria, parasites, and pathogens) but not such a great deal for you and your body.

Using the same thought process we used for leaky gut, imagine those smelly fellas getting delivered through your bloodstream to every body part, cell, tissue, gland, and organ. Do you think that might cause inflammation and potentially affect their function? If we have leaky gut, which causes infiltration, *and* we also have constipation or lack of timely elimination, which causes infiltration as well, we really have a double whammy.

Why be concerned with ridding ourselves of these toxins? Because if we eliminate them, they don't have a chance to contribute to potential gut and colon health issues. Consider colon cancer as just one example of a need for a healthy elimination process. Colorectal cancer, which includes both cancers of the colon and rectum, is the third most common cancer diagnosed in the United States (not including skin cancers). In 2016, it's estimated there will be more than 95,000 new cases of colon cancer (and more than 39,000 cases of rectal cancer) diagnosed according to "What Are the Key Statics About Colorectal Cancer?" from the American Cancer Society. Research published in *Pharmaceutical Research* in 2008 suggested that only 5-10 percent of cancer cases are due to genetic defects while the rest are linked to environment and lifestyle factors.

Cancer is a concern for all of us, but it doesn't normally develop all of a sudden. This means we have a chance to make changes that can potentially prevent cancer and other health issues from developing in the first place. One of the best ways to do this is to eliminate while also incorporating healthy diet and environment.

On the other side of the coin, we have diarrhea, which is not a normal way to eliminate either. Diarrhea is not just an inconvenience; it's a sign of a digestive system under stress. Often, the main causes of diarrhea are leaky gut and/or bacteria and microbiome imbalance. We usually have both since it's unlikely we have one without the other.

Americans have far too many issues with poor elimination—either constipation striking over sixty-three million people or conditions that have diarrhea as a symptom plaguing over sixteen million through IBS, Crohn's or Ulcerative Colitis, according to "Digestive Diseases Statistics for the United States" available at www.niddk.nih.gov/. What else are we known for? STRESS! We chase from one appointment to another. We have children's appointments, school functions and programs, sports activities, business appointments, etc. We have groceries to buy, doctors' appointments to make and attend, holidays and birthdays to prepare for, etc. What do we do during all this running and rushing? We eat poorly, our nerves get wound up or wired, and we hold it in the stomach. We find it really difficult to get time to slow down long enough to deal our job of elimination. When we do find the time, the colon doesn't always cooperate so we decide it takes too long and give up. Back we go to rushing. Thus, we end up with either diarrhea or constipation, and neither is a good thing. The effects of stress to manifest as poor elimination is huge, and it's showing up in record numbers for health issues today.

I'd surely work on stress relief and gut health to see if there isn't improvement before surgery or being committed to a lifetime of meds that disrupt other parts of the body.

Colorectal cancer is the third most common cancer for women in the United States, according to Centers for Disease Control and Prevention (http://www.cdc.gov). While we want to blame genetics, it's not only genetics. We may be predisposed, but one person gets colon cancer and the other person predisposed due to genetics doesn't. Why is this? It's called epigenetics—our ability to influence our genetic makeup. If cells are bombarded for years with excess toxins and invasive bacteria, it's bound to affect the makeup of those cells, yes? Therefore, if we don't remove toxins due to constipation, and they build up in the colon year after year, it's only natural we end up with a highly susceptible colon. (Remember, our conditions manifest in the most susceptible area.) This is one reason we say constipation and diarrhea are not just an inconvenience; it's dangerous to our health.

Regular Elimination

Before we get into thoughts of what we can do to help our elimination, it's important to know what is considered regular for the digestive system. You might already know you have issues or you might think you are a top-notch pooper when, in fact, you need to do a little improving. Let's review what's considered normal or regular, which is our desired result.

You should be eliminating at least once per day. For some people, *maybe* once per day is OK. Some people eat more *and* have a well-functioning system that results in 2-3 bowel movements per day. However, at a minimum, we need at least one per day. Going every 2-3 days? That's not good, and you may want to keep reading for some ideas to help with this. On the flip side, those with diarrhea issues might go 3-4 (or more) times per day, and that most surely is not good either (I suggest they also keep reading).

When we discuss normal stools, we also need to address what is *not* normal. *Abnormal* stools are:

- pencil thin (can indicate blockage or build-up)
- rabbit pellet type
- chunky with pieces of food in the stool (get those digestive enzymes with your meals)
- several lumpy pieces of stool
- diarrhea

What is considered a *normal* stool:

- one softer and longer snakelike-shaped stool, not broken up into hard pieces
- brown in color
- no large chunks of undigested food
- no extremely offensive odor (Even though all stools smell, a particularly strong, offensive scent can be a sign of parasitic bacteria in the stools.)

The above are some good guidelines for consistency of elimination. Now let's look at how we can help our body move things along in a normal manner—not too fast (diarrhea) and not too slow (constipation).

Keep Things Moving

The cause of elimination issues—all the way from watery stools to rabbit pellet stools to large, hard stools—can normally be a result of diet, low fiber, low water intake, stress, many medications, lack of movement (inactivity), an imbalance in intestinal flora, thyroid issues, or magnesium deficiency. The good news is there are many natural remedies to improve bowel function. Here are some ways to give support to our elimination process.

Ease Stress

Have you noticed easing stress is listed in *every* section on gut health? This is no accident. And although it's surely easier said than done, easing it must be done—or at least handling how we react to it. As mentioned previously, we will discuss some helpful ways to relax in a later chapter. But being mindful of your emotions and nervous system and the disruption and damage a stressed mind can cause is the first step to helping not only the digestive system but the entire body. A tense mind is a tense body, and a tense body contributes to a tensed colon that is just not designed to perform in an optimal manner. That's a fact. If the system that's engineered to move all the food, fiber, and toxins is stressed or tense, it can't possibly function properly. Stress equates to poor bowel movement function. Things such as deep, slow breaths when you feel overwhelmed, taking a short walk, and avoiding the people or situations that drain you can help you deal with life a tad better and relax the tense digestive system. Remember, we can't always control the situation causing the stress, but we can work on how we react to it.

Exercise

Most of us know there are multitudes of benefits to getting exercise or adding more movement to our lives. Two great advantages that apply to us in the digestion area is avoiding constipation by getting your blood moving and easing with that stress problem we just discussed. Movement is vital to circulation. Without circulation, our body literally cannot have the blood flow needed for body processes—including the elimination process—to function correctly. While exercise is good (and downright vital), avoid extreme workouts that raise our cortisol, stress the body, throw off hormone balance, and stress the digestive system. Think of it more as movement than exercise. Most of us tend to a have a habit of either not wanting to commit to an exercise program or we overdo it, which can be hard on a body already stressed.

Make your movement as easy as walks and some arm curls with light hand weights, which gets your blood flowing and heart rate up. Do whatever works for you—biking, treadmill, running, yoga—but the key is to make your movement program achievable. We need movement to get movement in our digestive system as well as to ease that load of stress almost every single person is carrying.

Fiber

Fiber is necessary whether you have constipation or diarrhea or normal stools. It has several uses, but one very important function is to absorb the bacteria and toxins to help carry them to the colon. It's gathering them up to protect us from remaining in our body. Now isn't that pretty darn nice of fiber to do that for us? When we think about the makeup of our stools, a good part of it is the fiber that absorbs the bad guys. This helpful fiber then comprises the bulk of our stools and moves along to carry them out of our body.

Fiber can come in many forms. One food that gets overlooked too often is quinoa. It has almost twice the fiber as other grains, is packed with protein, and is also gluten free. It's an excellent addition to help the digestive system. Always rinse it prior to use to remove any dust, and use it in recipes like oatmeal or as a rice substitute. There are loads and loads of great quinoa recipes online to help you incorporate it into your diet. Fiber also comes in a salad of greens, hemp protein, fruit, ancient grains bread, and oatmeal. You can also get it in sprouted chia or flax seeds (look on Amazon, Thrive Market, or a large grocery store).

Healthy Fats

Once again, we see healthy fats listed as something that will help our digestive system. For lack of a better explanation, let's think how important it is for things to slip, slide, and glide through and out the body. Obviously, this is far from a scientific explanation, but it makes sense that our entire body—our joints, our veins, our muscles, our intestines—need moisture and lubrication throughout. A teaspoon to a tablespoon of cod liver oil or flaxseed oil in the morning can do wonders for waking things up in the digestive system to stimulate the system to eliminate and/or to calm the system that might struggle with diarrhea. Incorporate your healthy fats but also make sure you are reducing the bad fats like processed foods, chips, crackers, etc.

Drink Lots of Water

Water is vital for hydration of the cells, but it is also vital to moving along the fiber we just discussed. In the course of a day, the digestive system secretes almost two *gallons* of fluids. Thus, it's important to drink our water. I like to fill three large glass bottles of water and set them on the kitchen counter each morning. If you work outside the home, take at least one or two of them with you to work. By the end of the day, all bottles should be empty. Make drinking water a habit that's ingrained as much as putting on your makeup or lotion.

Diet and Food

Obviously, what we ingest is important and also part of the solution to constipation or diarrhea. When you are grocery shopping or heading to the fridge for something to eat, choose an apple or other fruit, leafy greens, some prunes or figs, oatmeal. Try to remove gluten, sugar, fried and processed foods from your life. The trans fats in the oils from things like French fries, potato chips, and crackers slow down the system. They are also inflammatory, which can cause damage to the digestive tract and result in diarrhea for some people.

Avoid making meat the mainstay of your meals. Americans have a habit of wanting a big slab of meat on their plate rather than having meat as a side dish. Meat protein has some benefits (although most of these benefits can come from plant protein) but, as we discussed in the leaky gut section, it's also very difficult for the digestive system to break down. When you have meat, be sure it is from organic, grass-fed animals and avoid overcooking.

Magnesium

Magnesium is a vital mineral for healthy digestion as well as all body processes to help it relax and function properly. When we want help with relaxation both mentally and physically, magnesium is necessary. People with magnesium deficiency can't properly metabolize important fatty acids, such as EPA and DHA, which are vital to heart health as well as muscle, intestinal, and whole-body health. A good way to add magnesium is through magnesium-rich foods such as figs, avocadoes, leafy greens, pumpkin seeds, and almonds. Another good way to add magnesium is Epsom salt baths, which contribute to our absorbing magnesium through the skin. This can help with aching muscles or joints in addition to promoting bowel movements. Just like magnesium supplements, Epsom salt baths can cause diarrhea if we use too much so avoid getting carried away; roughly half a cup of Epsom salts for a bath is a good start and, if all goes well, you can increase if you prefer.

You might also consider using magnesium supplements. This is one of the minerals in such short supply in today's foods, it is unlikely we can get enough magnesium through our diet. Look for chelated magnesium supplements since a chelated form may help with better absorption of your magnesium as well as help avoid any bowel distress. There is also the option of transdermal (topical) magnesium in the form of gels or liquids. The advantage of this is the side effect of diarrhea may be reduced. Several good forms of magnesium oral supplements are magnesium glycinate and magnesium L-Threonate. Forms of magnesium to avoid are magnesium oxide, magnesium sulfate, magnesium glutamate, and aspartate. Avoid the last two completely. With some forms of magnesium, if we add it in too quickly, we can get diarrhea. Like all supplements and diet changes, ease into the amount used. An additional caveat is those with kidney disease should not supplement with magnesium without doctor approval.

Support Your Thyroid

If we have leaky gut causing inflammation to the thyroid, the thyroid may not be functioning properly. Since one of many thyroid functions is control of the urge to go, it may be the thyroid isn't doing its job to give that command. When we don't get the command to go, it's somewhat of a vicious cycle as we hold in toxins that cause inflammation and disrupt the thyroid even more. Help the thyroid support proper elimination by eating foods like those we have discussed, soothe and heal leaky gut, avoid fluoridated water, avoid heavy metals (metal fillings and vaccines), avoid gluten, dairy, and sugar. Hopefully, the thyroid will be in good shape to send out the proper signals to eliminate regularly.

Avoid Pain Medications

Medications can and do disrupt the body but pain meds are notorious for causing constipation. The less you can use these the better since we want to avoid the cycle of constipation causing toxins held in the body too long, which causes inflammation and contributes to pain. This causes many people to reach for a pain med that contributes to constipation that contributes to inflammation and contributes to pain, which leads to reaching for a pain med to start the cycle all over again. See how that works? It's a cycle we want to break if at all possible. Struggling pain is no easy task. The hope is as you ease inflammation, some of the pain will ease as well.

Avoid Dairy

Once again, we see dairy listed as a problem child in our digestion. This time, it's in our elimination section of digestive health and for good reason. The inflammatory, mucus-causing properties plus the hormones and antibiotics all add up to a drink that just isn't worth the downside of what it does in the digestive system. Milk was one of the first things we removed from our diet once we followed the path of natural health care.

Supplements to Help with Normal Stools

As mentioned previously, fiber supplements can be a helpful addition. They are a different form of fiber than our foods so don't assume using a supplement can replace fiber in your diet. And remember, when there's fiber ingested, you need to drink an ample amount of water to avoid clogging the pipes.

The aforementioned are a few of the basics steps to helping your elimination process. The key is to start with the basics to avoid getting overwhelmed. It's important if you aren't a regular pooper or you are struggling with diarrhea to know this is not normal, it's not healthy, and it's vital to undertake steps to have proper elimination. Let's have a quick review!

Sum It Up

To incorporate habits to help the body eliminate to eliminate:

- o Avoid stress.
- o Exercise and move.
- o Consume fiber and good fats.
- o Drink plenty of water.
- o Avoid pain medications.
- o Eat good foods and avoid bad foods (see below).

Cheat Sheet for Elimination

Yoga, Prayer, Meditation -NOT- **Rush, Rush, Rush**

- Exercise and movement

- Long periods of sitting

Foods with Fiber -NOT- **Processed and Disruptive Foods**

- Steel Cut Oatmeal

- Instant Oatmeal

- Leafy Greens

- Milk

- Quinoa

- Potato Chips & Crackers

- Prunes & Figs

- Bread & Pasta

- Flax & Chia Seeds

- Boxed Foods

- Fruits

- Processed Meats

Hydrating Drinks **Dehydrating Drinks**

- Pure Spring Water

- Coffee

- Alcohol

- Soda (Diet & Regular)

- Carbonated Water

Good Fats -NOT- **Bad Fats**

- Fish Oil

- Margarine

- Coconut Oil

- Canola Oil

- Flax Oil

- Soybean Oil

- Hemp Oil

- Vegetable Oil

• Butter & Ghee		• Corn Oil
• Sunflower Oil		

Good Supplements   -NOT-   Problem Supplements

- • Probiotics
- • Iron (can contribute to constipation)

- • Magnesium
- • Pain Medications (contribute to constipation)

- • Fiber Capsules

Chapter Nine: Calming Your Digestive System

This is the final topic regarding digestive health. Let's have a quick discussion on cleanses since they often come up in conversations I have with people working on their health. Cleanses have their time and place but often people struggling with their health will venture head first into natural health with a multitude of supplements and cleanse protocols. And that's wonderful—to a degree. However, we shouldn't use several supplements and initiate a cleanse or two without first eliminating some of the foods and toxins contributing to the problem. We should also introduce our soothing foods and liquids to calm things prior to major changes. When a person is struggling it's very possible his/her body isn't ready for a cleanse until soothing some of the body systems.

When I was struggling to help my gut health (let's be honest, it's an ongoing process), I got some very helpful advice from a natural health leaning doctor. His advice? Hold off on any cleanses until I had settled things down in my sorely stressed body. His thoughts were we need to work on at least *some* calming, soothing, and healing before we go dumping toxins from our organs into the stressed or sick organs that aren't in a position to handle them. Cleanses have their place and can be very helpful but approach them cautiously and wisely. Many people, when all else fails, decide they will turn to body cleanses to help with their health issues without first addressing leaky gut and bacteria imbalance issues. Many are even advised by our natural health professionals to do these cleanses. This isn't necessarily a bad thing, and I am not here to say don't listen to your health professional. However, there are many people buying armfuls of supplements determined to head home and get their cleanse going when perhaps their body isn't ready.

The problem with this scenario is most everyone struggling with health issues *has* a stressed body and overworked body systems. It's pretty safe to say for all of us, especially those with health issues, that over time we have absorbed and ingested loads of toxins that have built up in our organs. Let's say you used your hard-earned dollars to get some fabulous products for this cleanse. Let's also assume these products do their job of cleansing that organ. Awesome! You have cleared the toxins from that area of the body. But wait, where do these toxins go? They go into the bloodstream through the liver, kidney, gallbladder to be filtered and sent to the colon for elimination. If you have poor health and a stressed body, these organs and the colon will get overwhelmed since they won't be equipped to deal with or eliminate these toxins. The system is already on overload mode.

Therefore, the toxins circulate back through the body or out through the skin or begin stressing a different organ than the one cleansed. We have *retoxified*, which is stressing the body even further. Can you imagine your employer demanding you work fourteen-hour days until the point you get the flu? And imagine your employer saying, "You must work more to get over this inability to work hard." Now the employer demands you work twenty-hour days while you are aching, hurting, running a fever, and flat out exhausted. Instead of telling you to stay home, rest, eat chicken broth and take Vitamin C, you are told to work harder! This is an analogy on what we do to a sorely stressed body when we decide to do an organ cleanse without first helping the body get in better shape. What good will it do to release the toxins into our body if we haven't first learned and put into practice habits

147

that stop introducing *new* toxins through diet and personal care products?

Therefore, until you have calmed things down by cleaning up your diet, incorporated personal care products with fewer chemicals, soothed a leaky gut, *and* worked on proper bowel movements, a cleanse might not be the best idea. Love your body instead of placing unrealistic demands on it. Once you have done some calming and repair, then a cleanse might be in order.

Let's say you have worked on your gut health as well as decreased the number of toxins in your life. Let's also say you now feel your body is equipped to handle the toxin release from a cleanse. If that's the case, go for it. But be sure to choose high-quality products (no big box store brands), research, and/or get advice from a health professional. Go gently, gently, gently. We get tempted to want to get healthy—*right now*! Don't do it. Don't overload a stressed body. It doesn't matter if you want it done quickly or how tough a person thinks their body might be. The human body systems are only able to handle so many toxins at one time. When you are ready for a cleanse, it's normally a good idea to begin with a colon cleanse before other organs. It makes sense to start getting the bowels moving to eliminate the old toxins before adding in new ones from the stored toxins in our organs that get released from a cleanse.

If you are still working to incorporate healing habits and you feel overwhelmed by all the things you need to work on to help your body get stronger, hold off on the cleanse. Remember to take time to incorporate good habits first. Calm things down before trying to fix things up.

Concluding Thoughts on Gut Health

As we wrap up our lengthy discussion on gut health, know this. You do *not* need to have obvious gut symptoms, such as nausea, diarrhea, or acid reflux, to have leaky gut and/or imbalanced gut bacteria. All you really need are health issues or conditions... Period. These issues could be anywhere in or on your body or brain. Inflammation is a big culprit in many of our body issues, and a malfunctioning gut is a big source of inflammation. As we ease gut issues, we ease inflammation, and we hopefully ease health conditions.

Sometimes a person can feel as though small changes can't possibly make big differences and might not be worth the effort. I understand that thought process as I felt the same way. But remember small changes in daily habits add up over time. One small change made to a daily routine means you've changed something you do every day, seven days a week, fifty-two weeks a year. Eventually, those years become decades. Now does this one small change matter? Probably. And multiple small changes done over time can make a drastic impact. What if one of those small changes is something that might be causing major disruption for you or your child but you just don't know it until you try? If you never make the change, you'll never know.

Poor digestion, leaky gut, imbalanced gut flora, and constipation are common because of the modern lifestyle. Poor diet, stress, an overload of toxins in food and beauty products *and* a lack of educating us from our medical system have created a perfect storm for gut health. It might seem like bad news that you likely have some potentially big changes to make in your diet and lifestyle. The good news, however, is as a result of incorporating these better habits you have the potential to make major changes in your health issue *all by yourself.* Don't look at it as work; look at it as empowerment. Empowering yourself just comes down to the basics. If you learn the basics, you will support and maintain a healthy digestive system to help it function properly. Think of it as everybody has a job to do.

To recap, your digestive system's job is to:

- BREAK DOWN food.
- ABSORB nutrients.
- PROTECT the body from viruses and bad bacteria.
- SUPPLY NUTRIENTS to your cells, organs, and glands.
- REMOVE TOXINS from the body.

Your job is to help your gut do *its* job. Begin with the Focus Four:

1. RECHARGE Digestion: Rest the gut with easy-to-digest foods and digestive enzymes to assist in digesting.
2. REPAIR Gut Lining: Avoid leaky gut. Remove foods and factors that damage the gut.
3. RESTORE Bacteria and Microbiome balance: Support with probiotics and fermented foods.
4. RID Toxins—Eliminate to eliminate!

The practices for good gut health are repeated throughout our lists and discussion. Therefore, once you grasp the concept of healthy eating and lifestyle, you'll be equipped to apply these same practices to every other system of your body. You won't have to learn new complicated protocols for hormones or depression or anxiety. Our nervous system, bones, muscles, heart, thyroid, and hormone balance can all be supported, but we need to remember using the practices, foods, and supplements applicable to gut health to positively impact each part of the body.

The Takeaway

Ultimately, the body is an intrinsic machine with every body function, cell, and organ dependent on each other. No part of the body works or stands alone. This means taking care of all the body systems rather than just one area, but what is one super important area? The gut. Focus, focus, focus on your gut.

Isn't this a marvelous and fabulous thing to know? You have just learned that *you* have a huge influence on your health rather than relying on someone else to fix you. Ready to get started? If you're feeling overwhelmed because this is a lot of information, don't worry. Let's just start with the first week with Step One—a list of what I would do to begin helping the entire digestive system. These are what I consider absolute musts. Since I can't know each individual's issues, I'll start with the basics since, no matter what your issue, these should offer good support.

After you make these a regular habit, go back through the Sum It Up sections at the end of each chapter and cross off what you have incorporated. Then, make a list for your next steps, products, and foods you want to add. Keep doing this week by week until you are happy with what you are doing and, most importantly, until you see some change for the better!

Step One to Getting Started

1. Probiotics
2. Digestive Enzymes
3. Liquid Aloe Vera
4. Diet Changes
    a) Remove Milk

b) Reduce Gluten

c) Reduce Sugar

Use this above Step One list if you want direction for getting started. I'll list a few brands for the above starting list as suggestions below and a few places they are available, but there are loads more on the market. I offer these only as suggestions of ones I have personally used and liked. And remember to ease into the amounts you use.

#1) PROBIOTICS

Pick one. Get these on the Internet, health store, or large grocery store. Follow label directions. Use more than recommended if you don't see positive changes after a week or two of using them.

Brand	Where to Buy	Name on Label
Dr. Mercola	www.mercola.com	"Complete Probiotics"
ReNew Life	Target, Walmart, Walgreens, Amazon	"Everyday Ultra Flora"
Dr. Axe	www.draxe.com	"Live Probiotics"

#2) DIGESTIVE ENZYMES

Pick one. Get these on the Internet, health store, or large grocery store. Follow label directions. Use more than recommended if you don't see positive changes after a week or two of using them.

Brand	Where to Buy	Name on Label
Dr. Mercola	www.mercola.com	"Digestive Enzymes"
ReNew Life	Target, Walmart, Walgreens, Amazon	"DIGEST MORE"
Pure Encapsulations	Amazon, iherb.com, Swanson Vitamins	"Digestive Enzymes Ultra"

#3) LIQUID ALOE VERA

This is low in price, easy to use, and very soothing to the gut lining. It's a great way to get started. Make sure the package labeling states for internal consumption. I have used George's brand and had no issues with it; I also like that there is no taste. I only listed one other brand since most brands I found show additives and/or preservatives on their labels. Be sure to read your labels if you buy other brands. George's has less taste than Lily of the Desert, but both are good brands.

Brand	Where to Buy	Name on Label
George's Aloe Vera	Amazon, Walmart, Whole Foods	"George's Liquid Aloe Vera"
Lily of the Desert	Iherb.com, VitamineShoppe.com	"Lily of the Valley Preservative-Free Aloe Vera Juice"

#4) DIET REMOVALS

- Eliminate Milk
- Reduce Gluten
- Reduce Sugar

For the above list of Step One getting started, I've listed three products and three diet changes. This should give you a starting point!

I hope you've found these chapters on gut health helpful. Nothing has affected our health in our family more than changing our approach to diet and gut health. If you or a loved one has been or is struggling, I hope you will make the commitment to these changes and repairing the gut. Your effort will reap rewards.

Our upcoming chapters will discuss hormones, which is a hot topic for so many ladies. I will have what I believe to be very helpful suggestions for hormone balance. However, always keep in mind our discussion of how vital gut health is. There's a reason this has been a long discussion, and there's a reason it's the first in the health issues. It's the foundation for all other body systems including hormones. Nothing I suggest in the hormones chapter can be effective (at least long term) if the gut is in chaos or irritated. Therefore, start with the gut. Calm things down. Some of the hormone issues will calm just by helping the gut. From there, we'll have some other ideas for those pesky hormones. But first, work on your gut. You've come this far. Print out or write down the starter list above and begin!

The road of life is paved with flat squirrels that couldn't make a decision. I might change that final word from decision to commitment. Don't let lack of commitment make you indecisive and stop you from moving forward. Whatever your health situation, you now have the information and an opportunity to correct it *if* you believe in the ability of the human body to heal and *if* you take charge of what goes in and on your body.

Do not underestimate the power of what's on your fork, what's in your mind, and the removal of toxins from your life. Nothing will chase the medications and the body issues out of your life better than taking care of *you* with these simple gut health practices. Now let's turn the page and talk hormones!

Part Two: Hormone Balance

Chapter Ten: Hormone Imbalance

If I were a foreign country wanting to discreetly take over America, I would slowly infiltrate the governmental system to allow me to permeate the food system and personal care products. I would use the food and products to interfere with normal female hormonal systems and menstrual cycles, causing pain, mental health issues, lack of ovulation, and difficulties conceiving a baby—the very core of human life. I would use these same "weapons" to influence the health of the male population by reducing their testosterone levels, which would, once again, interfere with reproduction. People would actually invite these products and foods into their homes and bellies; they would even come to think they cannot live without my secret weapons of disruption. I would do it in such a covert way that nobody would make the connection between what I'm doing and the misery it causes. All the while, I would be taking away femininity, masculinity, enjoyment of life, and reproduction.

A person might think, "There's no way you could do this in a way nobody notices." But... I guarantee I could. How? Because it's happening in our nation right now! It's likely happening to *you,* your child, your parents, your co-workers and every other person you know. The most disheartening part of this scenario? Another country isn't doing this to us, but rather people who love us (they don't do it intentionally, of course), our food providers, health care, personal care companies, billion-dollar drug and chemical companies, legislators, and ourselves. Even worse, we might hear warnings of these invaders but ignore these cautions because we are really attached to these products and foods. And that's too bad. Because the above description of what will happen by continuing to use them is a very real scenario. Ignoring the warnings is the beginning of the end of not only optimal hormonal balance, but entire body balance.

Sadly, women's hormone-related conditions are common and escalating rapidly. Even if you have normal hormone balance, the life of a female can be challenging. We bleed, cramp, experience mood fluctuations, and endure labor and delivery. We struggle through perimenopause and then segue right into the lovely change of menopause with hot flashes and wrinkles. Hmph! Life can be a challenge with *normal* menstrual cycles and normal hormone levels. Now add the health issues of many females today, and our life becomes a great *big* challenge.

There is no question, as females, we have many blessings along the path of life. But lately, we have a record number with far too many struggles. We struggle with cramping. We struggle with severe PMS symptoms. We struggle with migraines. We struggle with anxiety and depression. We struggle with infertility. We struggle with Polycystic ovarian syndrome PCOS. We struggle with endometriosis. We struggle with severe bleeding during perimenopause. We struggle with severe menopause mood and hot flashes. We struggle with fibroids. We *struggle...*

And we are not alone. As testimony to the hormone imbalance present in our society, let's look at the statistics.

- Endometriosis affects 176 million women worldwide, and 1 in 10 females (10%) in the United States between the ages of 12-54 National Uterine Fibroid Foundation (www.nuff.org).

- Polycystic ovarian syndrome (PCOS) affects about 8-10% of women of reproductive age with supportive research available on www.womenshealth.gov shows

- 10.9% of women ages 15-44 have fertility issues (www.womenshealth.gov).

- 20-80% of women develop fibroids. This most often occurs during perimenopause according to the National Uterine Fibroid Foundation (www.nuff.org).

- By the age of sixty, one-third of women have a hysterectomy. Every ten minutes twelve hysterectomies are performed in the United States (http://nuff.org/health_statistics.htm).

- NUFF also states a hysterectomy is the second most common surgery among women in the United States.

- The average age for a young girl to enter puberty in 1900 was 14.2 years old. By the age of 8, 18.3% of white girls, 42.9% of black girls, and 30.9% of Hispanic girls have reached puberty, according to the September 2010, volume 26 of Pediatrics.

- The prevalence of postpartum blues syndrome is around 25%, and postpartum depression is around 10%.

- Women are 2.5 times more likely to take an antidepressant than men.

- One in eight women will develop thyroid problems during her lifetime, according to the thyroid fact sheet available on www.womenshealth.gov.

- One in four women in the United States in their 40s and 50s currently take an antidepressant cites The 2011 NCHS data brief "Antidepressant Use in Persons Aged 12 and Over"

These statistics are literally the tip of the iceberg if you research women's hormone-related health issues. They reflect the terrible price we pay for a lifestyle we aren't even aware can affect our hormone balance. It's a sad but preventable fact of being a female in our society today. Each of us is at risk to join these escalating statistics of hormone-related issues. I don't know about you, but I surely don't want to be a statistic for female issues. I don't like my daughter, my niece, my friend, or any female becoming a statistic—especially when it's so unnecessary and preventable.

Avoiding becoming a statistic is unlikely to happen if you see your doctor for help with hormone-related issues. The current practices for treating female problems in the medical system is, based on the numbers, obviously not curing us. The old adage says, "If it ain't broke, don't fix it." But current education and treatment for the female body in modern medicine *is* broke, and ain't nobody fixing it as evidenced by the number of medical buildings housing doctors' offices filled with patients. The overflowing doctors' offices prove and escalating statistics verify there's a problem in the approach to helping females. Our "help" comes in the form of synthetic hormones, injections, and surgeries removing our valuable body parts. This is not an answer to helping women with hormone-related conditions. This is getting sick care when what we need—and desperately want—is *health* care.

If you feel doubtful about the power of following natural health principles for healing, that's completely understandable. However, if you or anyone you know has been following standard medical care with limited results, I encourage you to consider natural health care. Because natural (commonly known as holistic) health care can be more powerful in helping you heal than all the surgeries, pills, injections, and procedures combined *if* you read, learn, and apply the information from this book and other research to your individual circumstances.

The Root of the Problem

One of the most important ways to help your situation is to look for the root cause of your particular health condition. In our discussion of hormone balance, we will detail the root cause in many of the female conditions we are seeing today. While we might think it would be normal to learn the root cause of health conditions from our medical doctor (it should be), information about body balance and healing rarely comes from our doctor's office in today's world. In our case with our daughter, Karly, zero of the information we will discuss to help with hormone issues was presented to us in any doctors' offices or hospital rooms. Over the course of fifteen years, she struggled with everything from uterine fibroids, heavy bleeding, severe cramping, blood in her stools, depression, anxiety, vomiting and panic attacks. We saw a tremendous number of doctors, specialists, and surgeons, but not one had a solution that removed her from even one single medication. Instead, six-month treatment therapy of toxic injections, as well as narcotics, birth control pills, multiple surgeries, antidepressants, and muscle relaxants were what she was given as the latest and greatest modern medicine. None improved her situation while her list of conditions and medications continued to grow. Consider the following potential causes that were not discussed with us. I suspect, if you are a female struggling with hormone-related issues, it likely has not been discussed with you either and any one of these could be a possible cause for you as well.

Studies show insulin resistance to be a factor in:

- Postpartum mood disorders (also caused by low progesterone)

- PCOS leading to infertility, according to the Johns Hopkins' Health Library

- Miscarriages in 27% of women (info from a 2002 abstract "Increased prevalence of insulin resistance in women with a history of recurrent pregnancy loss" from University of Tennessee Health Science Center)

- Behavioral changes including anxiety and depression, according to an abstract cited in Proceedings of the National Academy of Sciences of the United States of America's 2016 issue, volume 112.

Another big source of female issues is estrogen dominance with low progesterone. This is supported by Dr. John Lee's research as he cites (www.johnleemd.com) estrogen dominance/low progesterone as factors in a large number of female health issues including:

- Uterine fibroids

- Heavy bleeding during perimenopause

- Miscarriages

- Osteoporosis

- Breast cancer

- Thyroid dysfunction mimicking hypothyroidism

- Hair loss

- Infertility

- Endometriosis

- Early puberty

- Migraines

These lists *already* reflect some possible root causes readily available for your doctor to research and find, such as insulin resistance and progesterone deficiency, for many hormone-related conditions. By looking at these health conditions and their related causes, it's very possible there are substantial changes that can be made in the statistics for women's health issues through diet and toxin removal rather than medication and surgery. Since the above list mentioned insulin resistance and progesterone imbalance as causes in most of these female conditions, it would follow, at the very least, we should be told to focus on diet (since sugar is a big influence on insulin) and chemicals in our environment (since estrogen-mimicking chemicals in these products contributes to estrogen dominance) in our health appointments.

While we can be in and out of a doctor's office in fifteen minutes or less and leave with multiple prescriptions (with pages of dangerous side effects) for our health issue, we are rarely given any type of information on possible cause to our problem so we might heal the problem. Shouldn't we be made aware of the potential root causes and given suggestions on how to deal with things such as insulin resistance and estrogen and/or progesterone balance? Yes we should! All too often, however, we are shuttled in and out of the office, given a pain med, birth control pill, or anti-depressant, and sent on our (not so merry) way. How will that help us heal? The sad fact and harsh truth is that it won't. And we have statistics to prove it.

The medication we are handed can direct the body (even in ways it doesn't want to respond) or block signals (sometimes valuable symptoms as indicators to the issue), but a med *cannot* and *is not* created to heal.

Here is an example of the frustrating and upsetting type of treatment the standard female goes through today. I have a family friend whose daughter Kristine is in her thirties. About three years ago, Kristine had uterine fibroids. Why does a young woman in her thirties get fibroids? She shouldn't. I mentioned at the time of the fibroids to look into getting her progesterone levels checked since estrogen dominance with low progesterone is a common cause of fibroids. However, Kristine didn't do this because she got pregnant shortly after our discussion. Unfortunately, the pregnancy ended in miscarriage after twelve weeks. Since Kristine wanted to get pregnant again, I greatly encouraged progesterone testing to know her levels since low progesterone can contribute to miscarriage. Couple the miscarriage with her fibroids and the symptoms strongly point to low progesterone. Once again, Kristine didn't get around to checking her progesterone levels because she became pregnant soon after this conversation. She had bleeding in the first twelve weeks but retained the pregnancy and was blessed with a beautiful baby girl.

I cautioned her mother to be observant of Kristine's mental health after the baby since low progesterone is also a big factor in postpartum depression. Even females with normal progesterone levels have a major drop in progesterone shortly after delivery. Some women's bodies adapt and adjust back to normal levels, but often the ladies who struggle with low progesterone prior to pregnancy can have more difficulty adjusting back to normal levels. Sure enough, Kristine ended up struggling greatly with postpartum depression. She battled for about six months, trying to enjoy some of the best times with her daughter but often having this enjoyment interfered with by her depression.

Now, here's where things head south and, unfortunately, hers is not necessarily uncommon (one of many injustices to females and the reason for this book). Kristine made an appointment with her medical doctor looking for help with her postpartum depression. She requested progesterone testing based on my urging due to her fibroids, miscarriage, and postpartum depression all pointing to low progesterone. The result? Her doctor tells her he's never heard of low progesterone being a factor in postpartum depression. (Sadly, he most likely hasn't since this is typical of western medicine doctors.) He does *not* run progesterone levels and sends her home with a depression med prescription (which she did not fill). Kristine is now convinced her condition has nothing to do with low progesterone— because the doctor told her it didn't. This caused another three months of unnecessary struggling, lack of enjoyment of her baby's first year of life, and suffering more and more from depression.

Finally, she gave in to my nagging on progesterone and went to a chiropractor that ordered blood tests on hormone levels. In accordance with her symptoms, the blood tests show her progesterone levels are almost nonexistent. The chiropractor recommended a few supplements along with progesterone cream to hopefully increase her progesterone levels. Kristine was excited with her news and called to share the information. While I was happy that she found out her progesterone levels. I voiced concern about the cream she was given, thinking it may not be a strong enough amount of progesterone for her condition. However, it's better than nothing. Kristine used the cream as her chiropractor advised. Over the course of the next three weeks, she was not improving. Sometimes it can take a bit of time for the progesterone to kick in so all I could do at that point was encourage her to continue the cream or, ideally, go to a doctor who would review her records and symptoms to hopefully prescribe a bioidentical progesterone troche (a thin wafer containing bioidentical hormones that dissolves under the tongue) so she would get a stronger amount. Kristine had no idea who to call. Therefore, she made no doctor appointment and continued to struggle in silence.

Two weeks later, Kristine's mother called in a panic. Kristine had sent her a text saying the baby deserved a better mother and perhaps everyone might be better off without her. Now we have a major concern on our hands. Knowing her history, her extremely low levels of progesterone, and the progesterone cream was not a strong dosage, I searched to find a few apothecary/compounding pharmacies to get the names of doctors who have been known to use progesterone troches. After getting several doctors' names and calling to gauge attitude and likeliness to at least consider prescribing bioidentical progesterone in the troche form of delivery, I found a doctor for Kristine and made an appointment for two days later.

After Kristine's appointment, she called in tears. These were tears of happiness, not sadness, for the first time in eleven months. She informed me the doctor immediately agreed low progesterone at Kristine's levels were related to postpartum depression and also agreed she needed a strong boost of progesterone to help her with the bioidentical progesterone troche/water. She informed Kristine it was completely irresponsible that her former doctor had told her low progesterone had nothing to do with her depression (I completely agree), and she also concurred the cream was not nearly strong enough. Alleluia! Kristine had finally found someone who understood female health conditions; she was now on her way to feeling tremendously better.

While I would never discourage anyone from using depression medications since that is a personal decision, I most surely would encourage looking for the root cause of your condition. Had Kristine used the depression medications, she likely could have gone on for years living a subpar life and existing on pills because she had not addressed her low-progesterone issues. Even though she struggled greatly, she now has what she needs to feel better in a more natural way.

However, my next caution to Kristine has been that she needs to look for the root cause of her low-progesterone levels. Her likely place to start is with our gut health protocol from the previous chapter and the upcoming hormone balance checklist. Because, even though progesterone supplementation will likely help with the depression, the question remains as to why her progesterone levels are low. We will expand upon possible root causes of low progesterone later in this chapter. There *is* a cause for low progesterone levels, and Kristine cannot exist on supplemental progesterone long term, as it will be hard on her liver. She really should correct the cause of her low progesterone or the root cause will likely affect other body symptoms eventually. For now, things are under control. She feels strong enough to begin looking at diet, environment, and liver health to work with her body and correct her progesterone imbalance naturally.

The point of this story is that Kristine is representative of many women today. She suffered needlessly due to lack of knowledge on her doctors part. This is not uncommon on women's issues and it emphasizes the need for each and every one of us to learn all we can on our particular hormone related condition to avoid following the path Kristine followed. Hers is not a unique situation of needless struggles since I have seen this type of situation not only in our daughter's situation but in far too many other young women.

Looking at the statistics and the current mode of treatment makes it apparent it is up to each of us to take charge in our own health care.

A Simple Change

Females are a true miracle. We are blessed with beautiful, warm, fertile, loving minds and bodies. We are created with the wondrous ability to form a tiny human being. The human race would stop if we didn't have females to attract men, set up a home, and raise children. The complexities of the female body are wondrous but can also make life difficult at times. But just because our female body is complicated, it should not mean we are destined for struggles with hormone-related health issues. We should have energy. We should feel upbeat (most of the time). We should be looking at life as a glass half full rather than half empty. Most of all, we should feel like an attractive, energetic, and alluring female. That last part has been forgotten in today's world, hasn't it? And that's sad. Because too many women today do not get to enjoy life as my or my parents' generation did. Our struggles may have been money, establishing our family, job situations, or mother-in-law problems but rarely were our lives interrupted by a chronic hormone-related disorder. Today's women have all the normal day-to-day issues to face *plus* they have hormone issues manifesting into physical and mental problems. It's not fair, it's not right, and it most certainly should not be accepted as a way of life.

I want to encourage you to absorb the information we will discuss in this chapter to assist you in a more normal hormone balance and allow you to enjoy the life and female body with which you were blessed. I want you to have energy, sex drive, less pain, fewer emotional ups and downs, and fewer female issues. I want you to know it can be done. It *can* be done. And, honest to God, in most cases, it does not have to involve synthetic hormones, medications, injections, or surgeries. It can be done with changes so basic you may not be willing to accept that they can make an impact in helping your hormones balance.

I suspect if you are reading this book that you are more than a tad tired of gut or hormone issues (or both) as well as being shuttled in and out of doctors' offices when seeking help for what's happening in your body. You are not alone! It may or may not help you to know both my daughter and I have struggled with a myriad of severe hormone-related conditions. We have resolved our issues feeling not only normal but great—the best either of us has ever felt in our adult life. The steps we took will be listed for you so you don't have to deal with complicated protocols. Who has time for complicated protocols? Nobody.

If you read the suggestions I make and you make the decision to ignore these steps, I will feel not only sad but awful. Not that it matters what I feel because I will never know if you did or didn't continue. But I will feel awful for you because I *know* this information can be helpful to you to some degree. It may or may not completely turn your life around (although it might), but it can lead you to the information to follow or research further for better hormone balance *if* you give it a good, fair try.

Where I lose some ladies (especially younger ladies) is accepting something so simple can actually be powerful enough for whatever their issue might be. Getting used to being without some of the things they have been doing or using since childhood is also challenging. Normal, everyday practices or products in their world may be disrupting to their body and hormones. Some will decide there's no way they're going to avoid products they love or change habits they enjoy. If that is their decision, based on the numbers, it likely will commit them to a lifetime of female struggles *and* to standard medical practices of pills, injections, and removing body parts. No matter how you look at it, this last option is not a pretty future to face.

People resist change. It's a fact. We all do. But what if the things you change transform how you feel? What if you honestly believed food could be your medication to heal your body imbalances? If many medications originate from plants, then plants, as our food, surely can be powerful in what they do for our body.

You and I have a body that evolved from generations even prior to our grandparents. The cells, tissues, and DNA of our bodies expect and need food similar or the same as what our grandparents and their ancestors ate—food that it recognizes at a molecular, biological level. That type of food does not exist anymore. Well, at least not in the standard American diet. The fact is that type of food exists mainly in the organic produce section, the ancient grains bread that is rare and hard to find, and in meats from animals that graze in pastures. We no longer exist on food; we exist on food-like products. How can our body properly function with potato chips, brownies, sugared sports drinks or sodas, and boxed foods with a list of ingredients the body could never hope to recognize or utilize?

We are offering our body faulty information in the form of processed, chemically laden GMO foods. So when doctors say a condition is in your genetics, it very well may be that the condition is related to your genetics but in the opposite way we are thinking. The doctor may be saying your condition is related to faulty genetics when, in fact, your genetics may be exactly correct—inherited from generations of developing an optimal digestive system—but your genetics don't recognize or like the faulty nutrients of today's food. This particular paragraph may be key to this entire chapter. If we grasp the idea our food is incorrect rather than our genetics are incorrect when we have a health issue, it will make much more of an impact as to why we must change our diets or die. Die may sound a little harsh, but we can die while we are still alive; that's what malfunctioning, out-of-balance minds and bodies do. They die a little each day rather than truly living. What *if* we change our foods, remove chemicals from our environment, change our health, and really start living as we were created to live?

The healing ability in the constituent of a potato chip is a far cry from that of a carrot. And yet, since it's a pattern we have learned since childhood, we don't know how important choosing the carrot instead of the potato chip might be.

We follow the pattern we were taught since childhood to:

- Ingest the standard American diet
- Allow chemicals in our food, personal care, and cleaning products
- Accept the label of our diagnosed health condition
- Accept the prescribed medication without any instruction on healing

Hippocrates must be rolling over in his grave! If you read the previous chapters on gut health (and if you didn't, please back up and do so as we cannot balance hormones unless we have good gut health), you likely read about the hormonal struggles in my household. These struggles could have been avoided had we not been passive and if we had known the basics that ultimately weren't all that difficult for the solution we sought. I *wish* someone would have sat us down fifteen years earlier and explained to us that *what* we were eating, *what* we were using on our bodies, and *what* was in our environment was contributing to the cause of most of our issues. I wish they would have told us how standard medical practices for females were most certainly not the answer for most (if not all) of our issues.

Unfortunately, we were under the same belief system many women have today. We believed a personal care product on the store shelves must be safe. If food was on the grocery store shelf, it must be real food. Because

171

they were prescribed from a trusted source, we believed pills and surgeries were necessary to get better. We believed our doctors when they ran out of options and told us it was genetic. And we believed holistic or natural health was different and in no way as powerful as medication. We believed *all* wrong...

Nothing gives me greater pleasure than knowing by changing *our* belief system we no longer rely and live from doctor appointment to doctor appointment. We are down to only *one* doctor appointment for Karly for her yearly checkup and, for myself, zero appointments for four years. Do you think we might feel more than a little empowered? Yes, we do. Empowered and extremely thankful. The same empowerment I would love to see each and every female adopt. How did we get to this point? What did we do? What can you do?

Become Your Own Health Specialist

The very first thing we had to do was commit. Commit to questioning and, in our case, refusing all invasive tests, injections, and synthetic hormones. We had to accept that no matter how sick we were we could heal without these things even when medical testing was showing us evidence we needed the medicine or surgery. We had to refuse to succumb to the standard medical practice of the fear factor of what might happen if we didn't agree to these medical practices. By this time, our fear was stronger that if we continued these practices, life would continue to decline. Thus, we made the firm decision to commit to believing natural health could work and incorporated the information we learned to help ourselves rather than relying on the experts.

We made appointments with naturopath doctors to acquire and use only what we felt applied to our situation. No more blindly accepting what we were advised, even with natural practitioners. We started researching our particular medical conditions. What we did *not* do in our reading was go to the top medical websites that listed all the potential medical treatments to which we had already been subjected. Instead, we went to every holistic/natural health site we could find on our topic. We read not only opinions but actual research that supported those opinions. We learned what was truly a healthy food rather than trusting slick marketing on bags and boxes and, instead, making the bulk of our diet whole foods. We ditched the medical specialists who had focused on only one body system at a time. By reading, learning, and paying attention to whole body health as well as our body response, we chose to become our own specialist.

My encouragement to you is this: if we could learn and help our health to this degree, there is proof the ability is in each of us to help ourselves. While we sometimes need and want medical advice for extreme situations, for day-to-day health, we don't have to have a medical background. Sometimes I suspect we are better off that we don't because we are more open to avenues and alternatives that conventional medicine might dismiss or not even be aware of. Regardless of the arguments from medical professionals, you can't argue with results. So if a doctor, a nurse, or any type of medical professional challenges your desire to do things your way, don't back down *if* you have researched and you know it makes sense for your situation. Of course, if you have a sudden body or health change, you should visit with a medical professional. But for day-to-day female issues or conditions that have gone on for years with no improvement from medical treatments, it likely will be well worth changing direction to holistic health.

Changing direction may mean no longer relying on prescription medicine. Prescriptions of synthetic hormones cannot cure hormone issues. They control symptoms the body is intentionally sending out to you. Symptoms show the body has an imbalance, an invasion of toxins, and a disruption from some source. Look for what is causing the imbalance, but please do not tell your body to stop talking to you by thinking a symptom can be blocked with a medication and hoping the problem is gone. Even something as simple as taking an aspirin, Tylenol, or Advil for a headache should be something to avoid as much as possible. (Remember the gut health chapter that discusses the damage to the gut lining from these?) When you get a headache, first review what you ate (or didn't eat) that day, what fragrance products you might have used, and what stressful situation might be avoided. When we get in the habit of reviewing and asking why, we sometimes may have a revelation to a cause. If we pop the pill without stopping to ask why, we may never make progress on discovering the cause. Once we know the cause, we look to the solution by working with the body rather than stopping its communication to us.

Just as our body doesn't recognize the chemical messengers in today's average diet, the body also does not recognize the chemical messengers in synthetic, prescription medications. There's a reason each med comes with a list of potential side effects and reactions; the human body does not take well to body systems being forced into a response determined in a laboratory. Therefore, hoping a medication will cure has dismal odds. At best, the medication will block or disrupt symptoms and, at worst, contribute to new health conditions.

With that being said, you should never, ever, ever stop a medication suddenly. If you choose to remove or reduce medication, always wean slowly and check with your health professional (ideally, a naturopath, functional medicine doctor or natural health professional) on the steps to take to wean off the medication. Remember, the mindset of most western medicine health professionals may likely be to push you to continue the medication. If you are firm in your desire to wean off it, they should support your decision as long as it's done slowly with research to back your decision and the incorporation of healthier lifestyle habits. If they don't, it's time for a new health professional.

Once our health issue is labeled with some type of medical condition, we accept the label and assume it's ours to own. Once we own it, we become convinced nothing can be done. Remember, a condition is not a disease. There is a big difference. Bipolar depression and anxiety are conditions with diagnoses being a subjective opinion (albeit based on symptoms) of the one doing the diagnosing. There are many, many more health issue labels that are conditions—not a disease. This means the condition was created in the body, and the condition can be resolved by the body. There is a small percentage of instances where genetics make you more prone to that particular condition and in rare instances may keep you from improving but, in the majority of the cases, it's not genetics—it's lifestyle and toxin exposure. You may have the genetics to be predisposed to a certain condition, but epigenetics means we have far more influence over our genetics than we have been led to believe.

Whatever your level of hormone balance or imbalance, it's a rare female these days who isn't frustrated with the medical system's approach to female health issues. The more empowered we are, the more likely we might avoid at least some of the frustration, pills, and surgeries. When I discuss being empowered, it is so much more than a rah-rah cheerleader type of discussion. It's encouraging you to own your health, be the specialist of your wellness, say no to synthetic hormone prescriptions, and seek ways to support the hormone/endocrine system. When we switch our mindset to assuming it's within our power to heal rather than relying on modern medicine, we have taken one huge first step. To help you take that huge first step, I'm going to discuss what changes can be made to help hormones become balanced (or at least *less* disrupted).

Just as we discussed working on root cause for gut health, we will discuss root cause for hormone issues. To do this we, once again, have to remember the importance of the influence gut health has on hormonal health. Remember in gut health (we can't seem to get away from that topic, can we?) we discussed the inflammation that can come from an inflamed digestive system as well as the toxins allowed into our bloodstream to reach our glands and organs? *This* inflammation coming from a disrupted digestive system ends up affecting our endocrine system, the body system responsible for secreting hormones. If your thyroid gland, for instance, is inflamed due to leaky gut, it can't possibly correctly perform the functions it normally does such as regulating metabolism, energy, and nervous system functions like depression, menstrual cycles, etc. Now that's only one gland and already we have numerous potential hormone conditions from inflammation. Multiply and compound the rest of the endocrine system being inflamed (the liver, pancreas, pituitary, etc.) and imagine the potential interference of your entire female hormone/endocrine system and body from a damaged gut lining.

As you read, keep the following at the forefront of your thoughts: regardless of the female condition (and remember they very likely *are* conditions, not diseases), the practices we will discuss to incorporate into your life have the potential to greatly improve or resolve it. This includes

176

extreme cramping, miscarriages, hot flashes, depression, infertility, fibroids, thyroid conditions, hot flashes and more. Do not assume because tests show a blockage supposedly preventing pregnancy means you must submit to surgery or synthetic hormones—at least not before trying to reduce inflammation that may be causing swelling contributing to the blockage. Do not believe the only solution to fibroids and heavy bleeding is a hysterectomy—at least not before working to balance estrogen dominance and trying bioidentical progesterone. Do not believe that the newest and latest surgery to remove endometriosis cysts will supposedly stop the debilitating pain. (If that were true, one of Karly's four surgeries should have worked). It's always likely a test will find a problem somewhere. If you are having female health-related issues, there is obviously something wrong, and when something is wrong, it's likely to show on a medical test. This does not necessarily mean the result of that test requires surgery, medication, or injections at the end point showing an issue on the testing. The procedure at that point may not be addressing where the problem originates. What it does mean is there is a problem to address so we should address it accordingly.

Unless your situation is life threatening, before agreeing to any medications or surgeries, give the practices we will discuss some consideration. You can always consider the surgery at a later date, but you can't put a body part back once it's lasered, radiated, or removed. If inflammation is soothed or hormone disruptors removed, you might be amazed at what the human body can do to repair damage and come to balance. If the issue doesn't resolve, the surgery or medicine will always be an option.

The steps we'll discuss to feeling better are basic, but they are important. Often, the hardest part of taking that first step is to commit. If you don't like the thought of following the steps listed or giving up the things I suggest, think of the alternative, which would be continuing to feel like you are currently feeling. If that thought is not attractive, stick with me....

Chapter Eleven: Understanding the Endocrine System

All hormone-related health issues have at least one thing in common: an endocrine system imbalance. There is *always* a reason for this imbalance. We look to correct imbalances by incorporating the upcoming hormone balance checklist to ramp up our support to the endocrine (hormone secreting) system as well as supporting our gut health. The question then is what is an endocrine system? Most of us don't really want to learn all the glands or organs or the endocrine system. But we do need to learn enough to understand what's going on in our body so that you can help yourself.

What is an endocrine system? Let's take a quick look. While the nervous system uses electrical impulses to communicate, the endocrine system uses chemicals—your hormones—to communicate. Endocrine glands release more than twenty major hormones directly into the bloodstream where they can be transported to cells in other parts of the body. Our hormones are circulating throughout our bloodstream, coming into contact with all of the body organs. The only organ a particular hormone will affect, however, is the organ bearing the specific receptor contained in that hormone. This is rather like fitting a key into a lock where only a specific key opens a specific lock.

While most of us are familiar with hormone names, such as progesterone, estrogen, and testosterone, we aren't necessarily familiar with the endocrine system—the system in charge of secreting these hormones. Therefore, we tend to focus on an individual hormone when considering a health issue without being aware of the interplay of the entire system that secretes these hormones. One hormone-secreting gland or organ interacts with the others in a complex, intrinsic chain of events within the endocrine system and, ultimately, throughout all body systems. One hormone does not exist in a vacuum. Thus, when there is a hormone out of balance, the entire chain of hormones secreted by the endocrine system has something (coming in or being put on your body) that ultimately disrupts all, not just one. The disruption may manifest the most in the area that shows on tests or by our symptoms. Even though it may manifest in the area on the test result or in a severe symptom that does not mean this is ultimately where the problem originates. So rather than only focusing on progesterone, estrogen, or other individual hormone levels, we will also discuss the system secreting them—the endocrine system—the control center of our hormones and how to support it.

The Glands

Pituitary Gland

Located at the lower central part of the brain, this is considered our master gland since it greatly influences and controls the rest of your endocrine system. It is an important link between the nervous and endocrine systems and releases many hormones that affect growth, sexual development, metabolism, and human reproduction.

Hypothalamus

This is located in the lower central part of the brain and is the main link between the endocrine and nervous systems. It used the pituitary gland to link the nervous system to the endocrine system.

Pineal

Considered "Third Eye," it is located in the midbrain area. Unlike much of the brain, it is not protected by the blood brain barrier, which may make it more likely to be susceptible to metals and toxin damage. This gland is responsible for secreting melatonin hormone, which is involved in restful sleep.

Thyroid

Located in the front of the neck, this important gland secretes hormones that control energy and metabolism (think weight gain or loss), heart rate, nervousness, and a host of other functions. The thyroid gland tends to be one of the more easily inflamed glands in the body, and thus, it's one of the first to show up in medical tests with the answer being medications or cutting it out. Herein is a typical mindset with modern medicine practices. From a natural health point of view, does it not make sense that if the thyroid is inflamed, there is a reason? Lasers, medicines, or removal does not get rid of what inflamed it. Let's look for and remove the causes of inflammation, and let's leave our poor thyroid alone to do its very valuable job within our bodies.

Parathyroids

These are located on the back of the thyroid. These four glands serve a completely different role than the thyroid. They control the blood-calcium level. Calcium is important, not only for bones and teeth, but it's also vital to proper nerve function, muscle contractions, blood clotting, and glandular secretion. Like the thyroid, it's close relative, the parathyroid gets the brunt of inflammation and is prone to becoming a "sick" gland. Once again, the

181

answer is highly unlikely to be successful if that answer involves cutting or lasering it.

Adrenals Glands

These glands are located at the top of the kidneys in the middle of your back and are the busiest set of glands in the endocrine system since they secrete over thirty-six hormones. One of these is cortisol—our fight-or-flight hormone. Far too many women today have seriously stressed adrenals due to high cortisol from our stressed lifestyles. Now...if this set of glands is responsible for three-dozen hormones, and they become chronically stressed, does it follow your entire hormonal balance can be greatly affected? It sure will! This is one reason controlling stress and finding forms for relaxation is listed on the hormone balance checklist, which we will discuss in the next chapter.

Ovaries

Located in the abdomen, the ovaries produce our estrogen and progesterone, which trigger menstruation and, of course, are vital in reproduction. Estrogen controls the development of the mammary glands and uterus during puberty and stimulates the development of the uterine lining during the menstrual cycle. Progesterone acts on the uterus during pregnancy to allow the embryo to implant and develop in the womb. Mess with the ovaries (as our xenoestrogens most surely do) and we mess with a core part of reproduction.

Pancreas

This gland is considered part of the digestive system *and* the endocrine system. Within the endocrine system, the pancreas secretes the hormones insulin and glucagon to control blood sugar levels throughout the day. Since the pancreas is where insulin, the master of all hormones, is secreted, inflammation in the pancreas (sugar is a huge cause of this inflammation) will disrupt the master hormone and ultimately, all hormones.

Every one of these glands is important. Each is vital to proper body functions. This is why it is absolutely essential to do all we can to help a struggling gland or organ before we ever consider submitting it to damaging treatments or removing it via surgery.

Like the digestive system, in its own way, the endocrine system is a workhorse as far as the work it is expected to perform in the human body. If we look at body functions involved with the endocrine system, it might be easier to list what it *doesn't* control. The endocrine system is highly involved in the body functions of digestion, metabolism, weight, menstruation, respiration, sensory perception, sleep, excretion, lactation, stress, growth and development, movement, reproduction, and mood. Take a good hard look at that extensive list. Let's do all we can to soothe, support, and maintain this intrinsic system involved with our hormone balance. To do this, we look to ways to offer what the system needs. This starts with the items listed in the hormone balance checklist, which is coming up next.

Chapter Twelve: Searching for the Source

To help our hormonal issues, it's important to review our environment and personal habits as a starting point for the source of any imbalance. A good example why this is important is the thyroid hormone and gland. Dr. Mark Hyman, (an MD practicing functional medicine), likens the thyroid to being our "smoke detector for the fire going on in the entire body" (www.drmarkhyman.com).

What is bound to affect our glands (organs, joints, brain)? Chemicals. What do women do almost every single day? Apply chemicals through her personal-care products to her body. According to the Environmental Working Group (EWG), the average US woman uses twelve personal care products and/or cosmetics a day, containing 168 different chemicals. 168 chemicals. Not one. Not two. Not even five or ten. 168. This is *every* day—not once a week, month, or year. How is the body ever going to clear all these chemicals? It can't. Do we see the injustice of this to our body? We overload it with chemicals which wreaks hormonal havoc and our answer is to medicate, laser, or cut out the body gland or organ crying for help. We have makeup loaded with chemicals as well as shampoo, hairspray, and gel containing chemicals all used on the head that has blood vessels and capillaries flowing through the thyroid (and throughout the body). Women are five to eight times more likely than men to have thyroid issues (www.everydayhealth.com). While there may be reasons such as genetic components of male versus female, we can't ignore the amount of chemicals women are innocently exposed to daily through their beauty products. It's difficult to imagine why there aren't posters with red warning signs throughout our medical centers as well as warnings on every personal-care product container to try and stop this chemical infiltration by unsuspecting women everywhere.

What else contributes to inflammation that ultimately affects the thyroid? Leaky gut and sugar, which are both prominent in our lives. Between these and chemicals, the poor thyroid hardly stands a chance of functioning normally. Rightly so, tests will show it is not secreting the thyroid hormones at normal levels. And how could it? The poor gland is drowning, and nobody's throwing it a lifeline. What is the next step in this scenario? Prescription medicine or a laser and/or surgery to remove part or the entire thyroid, which ultimately commits you to a lifetime of medication. And all the while, the very source of the problem—chemicals, leaky gut, and poor diet—still remain.

Two statements I noticed while researching thyroid statistics from a prominent thyroid health site, The American Thyroid Association (ATA), state, "The causes of thyroid problems are largely unknown" and "Thyroid diseases are lifelong conditions that can be managed with medical care." First, I would beg to disagree that the cause is largely unknown—at least in the natural health world. We just discussed several potential causes. And second, telling us it's a lifelong situation to be managed with medical care is irresponsible at best, in my opinion. At the very least, the medical sites should mention (and, in my mind emphasize) the chemicals in personal care products. This is a big reason why, when researching a condition, it's important to get multiple points of view including—and especially—from well-documented health sites such as mercola.com, drhyman.com, or draxe.com rather than accessing medical sites that have the same information and mindset as your doctor's office.

The same principle we just applied to the thyroid is happening throughout the endocrine system to impact many of the body's health issues. The can apply the names of the glands, organs, and health issues from thyroid to the name of whatever a person's resultant health problem is at the time. The names have changed but the most common source remains: we ultimately come back to toxins, poor diet, and emotional health issues. The likely answer might be as simple as removing chemicals, addressing stress in our lives, and changing diet. Herein is the frustrating world we live in the American society and health system today. If we continue to accept the standard treatment, we accept that there is no cure. We no longer can continue to accept prescribed treatment while at the same time asking for sympathy and prayers. It's vital each of us stand up and decide we no longer choose to live the way of the average American. We must choose to clean up our minds, our homes, and our foods.

Finding the Imbalance

If we have an imbalance, how do we know? Symptoms are a huge indicator and, to me, one of the best indicators. Your medical professional can order a panel of hormone levels for you to get baseline levels or you can order tests online at sites like requestatest.com, healthonelabs.com, directlabs.com, or other similar sites. Insurance most likely will not cover your own tests, but sometimes it's worth it. My main concern with testing is to be cautious not to micromanage your hormones (or other body systems) as we just discussed. One hormone imbalance means all hormones are imbalanced, even if testing shows only a few out of range. If we only focus on one or two hormones or glands showing extreme levels in our testing with supplements or pills, we tend to forget the big picture, which is, ultimately, those out-of-range areas are a reflection of the whole endocrine system (and entire body). Therefore, we must remind ourselves, "Where is this inflammation coming from?" every bit as much as "I need to work on my thyroid." This is not to say we don't want to support the smoke detector (our thyroid), but we don't want to negate there is a fire. Therefore, while tests can surely be helpful, we must always keep our eye on the ultimate goal of putting out the fire through gut health support, proper diet, chemical removal and stress relief to support the entire body and all of its body systems.

It's extremely likely the source of *any* imbalance and the source for curing what ails you is somewhere in the list below on the hormone balance checklist. It may be found in one of them, or it may be found in all of them. The key is to know there *is* a source of imbalance that affects the entire body even if you only feel the results of the imbalance in one area. Avoid micromanaging in place of whole body managing. When we do this, we do not rely on the bad luck, bad genetics, or "if I supplement this one hormone or gland, things will be balanced" theory. No longer can we sit back and hope for improvement. We cause the improvement to happen by focusing on the items in our checklist.

Although the human body interactions and processes are complicated, caring for it does not have to be difficult. It comes down to this simple thought process: all health issues stem from a body system out of balance or overwhelmed. No injection, pill, or supplement can possibly heal or cure an imbalanced body bombarded by chemicals and poisons. The body heals itself but *must* be given the proper tools to do so. This means you have the potential to do something about it! Knowledge is *our* power in our lives and most certainly in supporting our body health systems including (but not only) our very important endocrine system—the system in charge of our hormones.

Hormone Balance Checklist

The following list is your guide to not only better hormone health but better overall health. Make a copy of your list, cut it out, hang it on your fridge, your bathroom mirror, your desk...wherever it might remind you of lifestyle habits to incorporate in order to live the lifestyle you (and every single female on this earth) deserve. This list involves the key to achieving energy, vitality, and that all too evasive hormone balance.

Here is your list. Make it a part of your soon-to-be balanced hormones, body, and life!

1. Minimize Sugar (Insulin is the Hormone Boss!)
2. Reduce Toxins/Chemicals
   a. Liver Care
   b. Xenoestrogens, add natural/bioidentical progesterone if needed
3. Reduce/Alleviate Stress
4. More Movement (but avoid strenuous exercise)
5. Digestive System Care (healthy gut)
6. Healthy Diet

The above list is short but powerful as far as help to the body. Below is a quick bit of information on the items on the checklist to help achieve hormone balance. We will dive into greater detail for each of the items after the quick overview of each of them.

Minimize Sugar

We will discuss ways to help balance insulin levels in our upcoming detail as a necessary means to achieving hormone balance. Insulin is considered our master hormone. When we consume sugar at the levels of most people today, we create major inflammation and our cell receptors also become insulin resistant. When the master hormone, insulin, is out of balance, it follows none of the hormones further down the chain like estrogen, progesterone, or testosterone can possibly be in balance. We do not have to be diabetic for insulin levels to be imbalanced and greatly disruptive in the hormones and body.

Elevated insulin levels caused by the bombardment of sugar and grains in our bodies can greatly affect our female hormones. Twenty-seven percent of women with recurrent miscarriages demonstrating insulin resistance in a 2002 case controlled study. Studies also show insulin resistance in females with PCOS (polycystic ovarian syndrome), according to the PCOS Foundation (w ww.pcosfoundation.org). PCOS is a leading cause of infertility with many females unaware they have this condition.

What could be a better example of disrupted hormones than insulin resistance resulting in recurrent miscarriages and infertility? These are only two examples of insulin-our master hormone- imbalance causing problems in the cascade of hormones. Imagine if you apply this information to each of the hormone-related conditions women experience today. Is it the entire solution? Of course not. The body reacts to a multitude of irritants such as chemicals, leaky gut, and high stress leading to high cortisol. However, imagine being made aware of the potential of insulin resistance as a possible cause for a woman struggling with this and other female conditions. If it turns out in a typical day she has a fruit smoothie for breakfast, a sandwich with two pieces of bread, a soda in the afternoon and an ice cream sundae for dessert in the evening—that will all contribute to sugar in the body. She may find by reviewing and changing her diet, she has the potential for great changes. But if she's never informed of the correlation, she would not know to review her diet. This is why looking for root cause of each health condition is where we begin when we want to improve. In this case—and many hormone conditions—insulin is one that should not be ignored.

We can ease insulin resistance by minimizing sugar and carbs, which can reduce hormone-related gland and organ inflammation and help with healthy insulin levels. This can assist our all-important master hormone to balance *and* take stress off the other hormones and body systems. Another great benefit of maintaining good insulin balance? It helps with appetite control, which obviously makes a difference in our weight gain or loss. We'll discuss that in the detailed section coming up.

Reduce Toxins/Chemicals

We will discuss the tremendous impact chemicals and toxins have on our hormone interplay as well as effective ways to greatly reduce toxin/chemical exposure. Our bodies are literally bombarded with chemicals and toxins on and in our body through the use of highly fragranced and chemically laden personal care, cleaners, and air freshener products (to name a few). These chemicals put major stress on the liver, the body's "clearing house" for chemicals and excess hormones.

Liver Care

High insulin circulating in our blood in addition to chemicals in our environment creates a massive assault on our liver. Why does liver care affect our hormones? Because the liver is a major player in filtering and eliminating toxins as well as excess hormones. It filters all that comes through the body whether it's swallowed, inhaled, or absorbed through the skin. The liver also plays a director role as it helps direct hormones to perform correctly in other parts of the body. One of the most important jobs of the liver, especially for our discussion on hormones, is that the liver's function is to remove or process excess hormones including (and particularly important for many females today) estrogen. Sugar and chemicals in the average female's day put more stress on livers than it can possibly handle and interfere with its ability to do its job to rid the excess estrogen, resulting in high estrogen and low progesterone—the stepping stones to a slew of female health issues.

Think of your liver as yourself on a day with company coming to your home. You are cleaning just as fast as you can. Meanwhile, the dog comes in with muddy feet, your little girl runs in from the sandbox leaving a trail, your husband brings his fishing gear into the living room to get it ready for fishing season (can you tell I'm originally a Midwest girl?), the air conditioning man wants access to the attic, your cell phone has six text messages and three urgent emails to answer and, meanwhile, your company called to say they are bringing their dog and sister with them. How would you react and would you handle it well? Perhaps for one time, but now imagine this goes on day after day, week after week, and year after year. That's how your liver feels. It can't possibly do the job optimally with the bombardment of "cleaning house" it needs to do. When the liver gets overwhelmed and loses its ability to filter and clear out the junk, our bodies retain too many toxins causing the glands, organs, and body to become inflamed and interfere with their ability to function correctly.

Xenoestrogens

We will discuss how to help reduce chemical and toxin exposure as well as supplementation to help with the imbalance they have created in many females. Chemicals are highly disruptive toxins that not only overwhelm our liver in its attempt to filter dangerous substances to your body but fragrance and other chemicals in our daily lives also create powerful estrogen mimickers called xenoestrogens. These powerful hormone mimickers can be 10 to 100 times more powerful than natural estrogen. Since it only takes a tiny amount of a hormone to have great effect on our body, a substance with the power of xenoestrogens can and does cause powerful reactions—and not in a good way—in the human body (both male and female). They contribute to estrogen dominance, which is literally fuel to the fire in the majority of the hormone-related conditions we see today.

If you struggle with estrogen dominant related issues, it may be necessary to supplement with added progesterone for potential relief to the imbalance of estrogen in relation to progesterone. There are far too many women suffering needlessly when they likely can get relief by using progesterone. There are products to support healthy levels of this hormone, but if you have severe female health conditions, you likely need more than support (maintaining). You would probably need supplementation (adding) of progesterone. This may mean getting an actual prescription for natural/bioidentical progesterone. This can provide great relief for many of our female hormone related conditions. Keep in mind adding progesterone is a potential *symptom* fix albeit an effective one. Therefore, as a symptom fix, it is not the long-term answer to the root cause, which is likely xenoestrogen-causing products, poor liver health, and diet. We will discuss root cause later, but for now, I mention supplementing with natural progesterone for those ladies unaware they may be able to get potential relief. The ultimate goal would be to use the information in this book to help you learn potential sources of the root cause of the problem so that you will hopefully no longer need natural progesterone supplementation.

Let's take a peek at the number of conditions often related to estrogen dominance and/or low progesterone (the two usually go hand in hand). These conditions may benefit from the use of *supplementation* (rather than a product that only offers *support* of healthy progesterone amounts) through added natural or bioidentical progesterone from your health professional. Conditions related to estrogen dominance and/or low progesterone :

- Miscarriage
- Fibroids
- Infertility
- Early onset puberty
- Cramping
- Excessive bleeding
- Migraines
- Postpartum depression
- Painful intercourse
- Vaginal dryness
- Loss of interest in sex
- MS

- Anxiety
- Depression
- Osteoporosis
- PCOS
- PMS
- Hot flashes
- Menopause mood issues
- Irregular menstruation

We will discuss how and why progesterone may be beneficial in the detailed section on this subject later in the hormones section. For now, be aware there may possibly be potential relief without drastic treatments.

Reduce/Alleviate Stress

The number one area I recommend to begin in this area is to be mindful of stress that leads to high cortisol levels. Far too many women lead stressful lives that result in stress on the entire body. Of particular concern with our females today are the elevated cortisol levels, which ultimately place an extreme burden on the endocrine (think adrenal and thyroid glands), nervous and digestive systems, as well as interfering with our progesterone synthesization as well as our all too necessary healing and restorative sleep. Incorporating stress-relief methods, learning to control how we react to stressful situations, and doing all we can to reduce stress can have major impact on hormone (and body) balance.

More Movement

We will later discuss the benefits of circulation as well as some simple tips to increase it. Circulation is vital to help our overloaded liver, our lymph system (lymph glands are in our thyroid), and proper function of all body systems. Make it a goal to fit twenty minutes of activity in as many days as possible. We simply are not moving enough, and circulation is vital to proper gland and organ function. Movement or exercise is important for circulation, mental health, and disposal of toxins. While movement is necessary for good health, we will discuss the need to avoid intense workouts that can result in high cortisol and thus, stressed adrenals.

Digestive System Care

We will have a short summary of how the digestive system interacts with other body systems to affect hormone and whole body balance. Hopefully, we should not have to spend too much time in this category since we have an entire section on this subject. What I do want to emphasize is the importance of reading the previous chapter as well as incorporating the steps listed in the gut health chapter, into your life. We cannot possibly balance hormones if we have an inflamed gut. Inflamed gut leads to an inflamed endocrine system. An inflamed system will not secrete proper hormone levels. We want to soothe and support the whole body versus zeroing in on one or two glands and hormones or systems. To do this, we need a healthy, well-functioning digestive system.

Healthy Diet

We will discuss the foods to avoid as well as some to include in your daily diet so that your body gets a break from damage and inflammation. You are what you eat is so much more than a cliché. Better food choices lead to better hormone (and whole body) health. Potato chips, boxed or bagged cereal, bagels, white bread, and commercial milk are not body-nurturing and supporting foods. They are inflammatory foods that *will* lead to body inflammation, which *will* lead to gland and hormone disruption. The average American diet lacks nutrients and contains far too much sugar and damaging chemicals that compromise the gut lining. When we offer healing nutrients and foods, the body lets out one great big sigh of relief and can get to work on coming to homeostasis (balance).

There you go! Your hormone balance checklist is listed above. This is a list of areas that can make big changes to the balance in your endocrine system and thus, your hormone balance! *Whatever* you do at this point in your reading, please do not look at this list and tell yourself it's too basic and not powerful enough. If you do, your odds of balanced hormones will likely reduce exponentially. This list really can work. It didn't just work in our case; although these practices brought results that were it was a small miracle for my daughter and myself as well as a multitude of women I have counseled. Our lives have been changed more for the better than we ever could have imagined. And it can work for you. Choose the things on the list you *can* live with for now. None of these involve a big time commitment or huge expenses. Even if they did, what price would we put on good health and feeling great? Perhaps you already do some of these things and, if so, good for you. The key now is to continue with the ones you are doing and add in those you aren't. What matters more than anything on this list is your mindset and your commitment. Start with *some* on the list but vow to incorporate *all.*

Chapter Thirteen: Minimizing Sugar

We briefly discussed each of the items on the checklist, and we will now delve into further detail on each of these topics for a better understanding of how each of these contributes to hormone related conditions and to help us find the root cause. Understanding the how and why enables you to know what your part will be in working to alleviate or resolve the condition.

The first on our checklist is minimizing sugar to avoid high insulin levels that lead to insulin resistance in our cell receptors. I know insulin doesn't sound too exciting but in its contribution to either disrupt or ease hormone issues, it *is* exciting. It's the first area we addressed for both Karly and myself in dealing with our hormone imbalances. We tend to think of insulin as a diabetes issue (which it is) and something our older aunt, uncle, or grandparent needs to be worried about (which it was). About fifty years ago, you would have been right; it was an older person's condition. The average female (especially younger ladies) does not place a high importance on insulin levels nor do they even consider it something to be concerned with. If we do worry about it, it's in relation to trying to lose weight.

Insulin levels are so much more than just weight control, and they most surely are no longer only an older person's concern. The fact that this used to be mostly an older person's concern may be a big reason why so many doctors have not zeroed in on it as a cause for younger ladies with their hormone-related conditions. If learning about insulin isn't your favorite way to spend your time, it's an important part of getting to root cause so be patient as I truly believe every single female needs to be made aware of this area of her life. It's influence on our hormone balance is the reason I have made it the very first item on our hormone checklist. I guarantee it *is* something the average female should be concerned with regardless of whether they are one year old or one hundred years old, particularly in today's environment and lifestyle. If I do a decent job of conveying the importance of this area, I believe you will consider learning about insulin time well spent.

Is sugar intake (thus insulin levels) a concern for you and for the average American? Check the statistics. According to the Harvard School of Public Health, more than 70 percent of Americans eat at least 22 teaspoons of added sugar daily yet The American Heart Association (AHA) recommends no more than 6 teaspoons (25 grams) of added sugar per day for women and 9 teaspoons (38 grams) for men. Six teaspoons is the recommended amount and yet we average twenty-two? That would mean the average female is consuming almost four times the recommended amount. Truth be told, we don't really need *any* teaspoons of sugar since we get all we need, even in healthy diets.

No matter your gender, the American Heart Association's article "Sugars 101" claims one single 12-ounce can of Coca-Cola goes over the maximum sugar allowance for the day. This statement is regarding adults. Now imagine a child and consider how often they drink a can, bottle, or a glass of soda at a fast food restaurant. Factor in those children (or yourself) that do not realize a glass of orange juice has a similar amount of sugar in it, and we can see the way sugar makes its way into our body. This amount of sugar in our body, especially in a young body, is literally a path toward health destruction.

Discussing insulin is not the first on our checklist by coincidence.

It's #1 because sugar has become an overlooked, invasive, destructive factor in insulin-resistance levels and, ultimately, hormone balance. Since insulin is considered our master steroid hormone, it follows that no other hormone can be in balance if the guy at the top of the chain is "out of line or disrupted."

In Chapter Ten, I listed studies linking insulin resistance to miscarriage and infertility. Now let's consider mental health and sugar intake. Insulin is also produced in the brain so do you suppose if you have improper levels of insulin in the brain that it might affect mood, anxiety, and depression? Consider the following from the Joslin Diabetes Center's 2015 article "Insulin Resistance in Brain, Behavioral Disorders":

> Genetically modifying mice to make their brains resistant to insulin, the Joslin scientists first found that the animals exhibited behaviors that suggest anxiety and depression and then pinpointed a mechanism that lowers levels of the key neurotransmitter dopamine in areas of the brain associated with those conditions. This is one of the first studies that directly shows that insulin resistance in the brain actually can produce a behavioral change.

Miscarriage, infertility, depression, and anxiety are all linked to insulin resistance with insulin resistance a result of high sugar and carbs intake. These are most surely not the only hormone-related health conditions linked to sugar/carb intake and the resultant insulin resistance. Earlier, I mentioned we would connect the dots of female hormone-related conditions to diet as well as toxins in our environment. We are barely into this chapter and already we can see a big potential factor—insulin levels from high sugar and grains intake—that has likely never been brought to your attention at the doctor's office if you struggle with one of these conditions. Let's factor in the disruption of the chemicals/toxins on our liver health then multiply the hormones cascading from this disruption of our insulin (estrogens, progesterone, testosterone, DHEA, etc.) that ultimately are influenced by insulin imbalance. Does it make sense the destructive impact these would have on literally any female (and male) condition?

Some health professionals have become aware of the link between insulin and PCOS. Unfortunately, we are back to the synthetic answer as they tend to prescribe metformin, an insulin-related drug. Remember, medication is the only answer at their disposal thanks to our pharma-influenced health care system. Giving you a talk on watching your sugar intake and sending you home with the advice to curtail sweets and carbs is unlikely to happen. Thus, the flaw of today's system: why would you need a drug to manipulate your insulin when changing your sugar and carb intake would do the same thing naturally (and safely)? Taking a medication but doing nothing to change the root cause of your diet is a sure path to bigger health issues down the road.

Disrupting the Insulin Hormone

Why does our insulin hormone get disrupted and out of balance to create insulin resistance? Let's look at how sugar and insulin interact in our bodies. The average adult has about one gallon of blood in his body with the amount of sugar in that gallon being only one teaspoon of sugar (or less). The body works hard to avoid any more sugar than one teaspoon in the blood at all times. If your blood sugar level was to rise to just one tablespoon, you have a risk of going into a hyperglycemic coma with the risk of dying. To avoid this, your body has a multitude of intrinsic processes it performs to prevent excess sugar levels. (Your body is not a big fan of coma and death.) A huge part of this process is to produce the insulin hormone to maintain proper sugar levels in the blood.

When you consume foods high in sugar, grains, or carbohydrates, you typically have a rapid rise in blood glucose. To regulate the levels in the blood due to this rise, your pancreas secretes insulin into your bloodstream to help pull the sugar from the bloodstream and store it in your cells. This lowers the sugar amount in your blood to prevent coma and death. However, the insulin secreted into the bloodstream can quickly drop your blood sugar level. While this may be good for avoiding death, it can also swing you the other way, resulting in a drop that causes intense cravings for more of the same disruptive hormone in carb-rich and sugar-laden foods. You are now at that point many people experience where you will eat most anything in sight, including the arm off of your chair. Now is really *not* the best time for resisting sweets. You are starving (actually your cell receptors are screaming for more sugar), and you are absolutely going to eat what makes you feel better.

Therefore, as we consume a diet consistently high in sugar—whether it's processed foods, soda, juice, even fresh fruit as well as grains in the form of bread or pasta—your blood glucose (sugar) levels will respond accordingly and ultimately remain elevated in your blood due to the constant need for you to feed them. This elevated high level causes the pancreas to work overtime, sending out more insulin in an attempt for the insulin hormone to remove the glucose/sugar from your blood. Over time, your body cells that normally receive the insulin hormone become insulin resistant or desensitized to it. It's somewhat like your best friend stopping by for a surprise visit. The first time or two, you are delighted to see her. After a while, it becomes inconvenient and, if she continually stops in, downright disruptive. The same applies to insulin constantly knocking at the cell door wanting to drop off excess glucose it is removing from your bloodstream. After a while, the cell has welcomed all the glucose it can handle (and normally more). The cell is overloaded with glucose from insulins deliveries—the cell becomes resistant to opening the door. This requires your overworked pancreas to secrete more and more insulin so it has more power to "knock louder and more forcefully" in an attempt to get the cell to open the door to insulin and allow it to drop off the glucose from the bloodstream and store it in the cells. Medication will attempt to curtail the amount of insulin secreted when, in essence, the problem isn't insulin; it's the high sugar amounts in the blood. Lowering the insulin attempting to remove the excess glucose from high sugar intake works against the body. We *need* our insulin to continue its job of removing the glucose, but what's most important is that we also need to ease the sugar in our bloodstream. The root cause isn't a high insulin problem; it's high sugar intake.

Your cells are overloaded with glucose/sugar. Their best way to deal with this is to store it in fat. This is one reason why losing weight isn't always about calories as much as what *type* of calorie. Sugar calories are guests welcomed only in the area undesirable to us—the fat cells. The more sugar overwhelms the body, the more fat cells need to be created to deposit the unwelcome guests. Over time, your cells become insulin resistant, and eventually, you can become diabetic. The worst part is that you don't *know* you are insulin resistant because, as someone who has no reason to suspect insulin issues, you've never considered it as a potential problem-especially younger females. But the health effects of this elevated blood sugar/insulin cycle begin to occur even before insulin resistance sets in.

This much I can almost guarantee: if you have hormone issues, you likely have some level of insulin-resistance issues regardless of whether your tests show your ranges are normal. Therefore, if you have hormone-related problems, reduce sugar intake and watch body response as the best indicator. If you did test and you found elevated insulin levels, what would you do? I would hope you would reduce sugar and carbs. Getting a test for a baseline value may be helpful but rather than waiting for a test to convince you, look to your symptoms and do an honest review of your carbs/sugar intake. Be proactive (not reactive), and cut your intake just like you would if you ran a blood test that showed elevated levels. You can do it now, or you can do it when the pancreas gives up trying to secrete insulin at continual high levels in its attempts to control the excess glucose in your blood. At that point, the repair would be much more difficult and time consuming than being proactive and avoiding the damage.

In his 2013 article "How Sugar Can Become Toxic," Dr. Mercola states, "If you received your fructose only from vegetables and fruits (where it originates) as most people did a century ago, you'd consume about 15 grams per day. Today the average is 73 grams per day, which is a nearly 500 percent higher dose..." From 15 grams to 73 grams? How did we get so far from eating correctly? Even worse, those grams in our grandparents' day normally included antioxidants, nutrients, and fiber in the form of fruits. The majority of our sugar intake is soda, sweet treats, or processed grains with little to no nutrition value.

Increased insulin resistance contributes to chronic inflammation in your body, and inflammation (as we discussed extensively in the gut health section) is the hallmark of most health conditions and disease. Over time, sugar causes continued stress on the liver (where our hormones are synthesized and processed) as well as insulin resistance. "Over time" in our grandparents' day normally occurred near the age of seventy. Our intake in today's society starts at high amounts from a young age. This sugar and carb intake not only continues, but consumption increases through the years when the cell receptors demand more sugar as they become addicted to the rush. If you ignore the demand, your body will feel completely "off" until you give in and supply those addicted cell receptors with what they demand... sugar. Ultimately, due to this high intake, what used to be a concern in old age has now become a young female concern (as well as older females and males) often without their awareness to the issue. When it becomes a health issue does not necessarily mean you are at diabetic levels...yet. Therefore, you remain unaware it exists other than the hormone imbalance symptoms that may be a message from your body about the insulin resistance. Unfortunately, if you or your doctor don't consider insulin issues, you might get diagnosed as having something completely different such as a thyroid or pituitary issue and given meds for those glands rather than the simple fix of reduced sugar intake.

Supporting healthy blood sugar levels became our main focus on the road to better health for our daughter's daily protocol. Even though no doctor or test ever indicated this should be her starting point, it was the top area to start in her diet as she began weaning from her twelve medications. This focus on avoiding sugar and carbs, eliminating chemicals/toxins, and supplementing with progesterone were our starting points. I would suggest for any female struggling to remove sugar as much as possible to increase the odds of seeing positive changes to her hormone balance.

The Danger of Sugar

Hormone problems might seem as they happen suddenly but, in reality, they manifest over time. The inflammation and chemicals build over years of using products with chemicals and ingesting sugar and grains as a normal part of the everyday diet. The body does a fabulous job of sorting and putting away any overloads for years, sometimes decades. So, we don't think or know we have inflammation and hormone issues waiting to emerge.

As PreventDisease.com claims, "The average child today by the age of 8 has had more sugar than the average person did in their entire lifetime just one century ago!" This is a sobering thought for our children. We need to change our children's reward system if we are going to change the chaos to our hormones, endocrine system, and overall body support. This is a cold, hard fact. If we don't change our children's diets and stop rewarding with sweets, we are setting them—and ourselves—up for a lifetime of potential health conditions. Unfortunately, sugar is a big ingredient in almost every single processed and packaged food including baby formulas. Research shows that, literally, the cell receptors that crave highly addictive drugs, such as cocaine, are the very same receptors that crave sugar, as noted in the 2007 article "Intense Sweetness Surpasses Cocaine Reward." This research claims sugar is ultimately even more "rewarding and attractive than cocaine" (www.ncbi.nlm.nih.gov).

Sugar is every bit of a real addiction as drugs! Who knew *that* information when they were handing you a soda or cookie for your treat when you were a little girl? As a parent, we love to see our child's eyes light up when we offer them treats like ice cream, suckers, cookies, cupcakes, or grains like bagels, chips, or crackers. We may love their reaction, but it's sobering to think what else lights up as a result of the insulin-disrupting sugar in the treat; every cell and tissue in the body experience some degree of inflammation leading to disruption and, as the years go by, ultimately hormone-related health conditions.

Help you and your child get back to the days when sweets were reserved for special occasions, not an everyday reward and habit. Remember the end result if sugar or carbs remain part of your everyday diets. You will have to decide what is more important, a temporary rush when you eat and pleasing your child with sugar or watching the results further down the road of a sugar-laden diet? The sugar rush is temporary; the damage it does to hormone levels (and overall health) is long lasting.

You may also think this can't possibly make enough difference to really affect your major hormone issues.

I cannot emphasize the following any better than Dr. Mercola, one of my all-time favorite natural health proponents. His comments regarding sugar in relation to our American diet are spot on. In the 2011 article "Eliminate This ONE Ingredient and Watch Your Health Soar," he says:

> Remember, the average person is consuming 1/3 of a pound of sugar EVERY DAY which is five ounces or 150 grams, half of which is fructose or 300 percent more than the amount that will trigger biochemical havoc. Remember, that is the AVERAGE; many consume more than twice that amount... [Sugar is] loaded into your soft drinks, fruit juices, sports drinks, and hidden in most processed foods—from bologna to pretzels to Worcestershire sauce to cheese spread. Even most infant formulas contain the sugar equivalent of one can of Coca-Cola! To put the US sugar consumption into further perspective, based on USDA estimates the average American consumes... about TWO TONS of sugar during their

lifetime. Try to imagine that amount. Two tons! Is it any wonder then that the United States is the fattest of thirty-three countries, with a whopping 70 percent of Americans crowding into the overweight category? No, there can be no doubt whatsoever that this is a direct result of excessive sugar consumption, and the fact that this sugar-rich diet also fuels a number of deadly diseases is another no-brainer. Yet conventional medicine keeps ignoring the basics, seeking to find magic solutions in the form of a pill. Do yourself and your family a huge favor, and educate yourself on the health effects of sugar instead, because the truth is, simply making this ONE lifestyle change—drastically reducing your sugar consumption—is the "miracle cure" everyone is seeking!

Over time, high sugar intake, as Dr. Mercola states, is literally abuse. It eventually causes damage to our chemical messengers, our hormones. Please note he does not say it causes a little bit of a problem. He uses the words "biochemical havoc," a powerful but very appropriate phrase. The foundation may have been laid years ago for a lifetime of sugar disruption, but you can change the foundation by transforming your diet for a more balanced endocrine system, which results in more balanced hormones. Suggested changes in diet and food tips to help avoid or reduce insulin resistance will be listed in the healthy diet section at the end of this section on hormone balance. Please review and incorporate those tips; it will be well worth your time to help avoid some of the pitfalls I encountered when first venturing into the confusing natural health foods arena.

The Power of Change

While I can explain why you should change, there is obviously nothing I can list here to make the changes for you. We have repeatedly discussed the potential damage of insulin resistance to not only your hormone health but your overall health. Ultimately, you are the one who says "no more" on the sugar- and carb-laden diet. Nothing you could do would be a bigger gift to yourself and your children than to make this decision and take the needed steps. Removing carbs and sugar may seem overwhelming (and it is to a degree, especially at first). But hang in there because you know you are making a fabulous, positive step. You can either go whole hog, or you can ease off on the bad foods slowly. I found going whole hog easier, but do what works for you.

I also pick my poison. I am good 90 percent of the time, and 10 percent of the time I indulge if I want. There are natural health people who will say absolutely no to any of the bad stuff. That, of course, is your decision. We are all snowflakes—similar in our makeup but different in our pattern. Even though I have found what works for me, you will need to watch body reactions and gauge accordingly as far as what works for you. If sugar and carbs throw you into a tailspin, you obviously can't (or at least shouldn't) have them.

I have had people tell me if they remove what we label as bad foods or ingredients, there is nothing left to eat except lettuce, which surely doesn't satisfy. I get that. But here's where the road forks. You can have that mindset and keep filling the hole accordingly or you can go with the mindset that you *will* find foods to satisfy you. I won't lie. The first few days, even a couple of weeks, are tough because we have addicted cell receptors begging for mercy in the form of sugar or carbs. But hang in there. You will find foods that are healthy and yet filling. It will take some time investment, but nothing good ever comes without effort. Many people end up feeling so much better that they now enjoy grocery shopping and getting creative with their meals. After a couple of weeks, you may be surprised how your nose actually turns up at a brownie or loaf of white bread. It might take longer than a couple of weeks (or it might not), but if you really do adopt the healthier diet, you will eventually stop craving and literally be turned off by the unhealthy foods.

All the books, seminars, videos, or articles in the world cannot do for you what needs to be done. Stop lifting the hand to the mouth with unhealthy foods. While that may sound harsh, it's true. The same applies to each and every one of us. Food, stress reduction along with chemical/toxin avoidance are the beginning steps to change our health. Supplements are great. Acupuncture, massage, and chiropractic treatments are awesome. Most of the natural health modalities on the market have some good benefits. But nothing changes our health like ingesting decent food.

Your insulin hormone is your friend on the road to hormone balance. Where it no longer becomes your friend is when you abuse it with continual sugar and grain assaults. Back off on the sugar, eat healthy, apologize to insulin, and become friends again. Insulin is one of the most powerful, effective means to hormone balance, which makes it well worth extending the olive branch.

Chapter Fourteen: Reduce Toxins/Chemicals

The effect of chemicals and toxins is a key factor in hormone disruption, and it is next on the hormone balance checklist. We will discuss the influence of chemicals in causing damage and creating powerful estrogen mimickers called xenoestrogens. We will also cover what products contain chemicals and ways we are exposed to these chemicals so that we can move our focus to xenoestrogens and the use of (natural) progesterone.

Chemical Onslaught

The Environmental Working Group (EWG) recently released data from tests on ten blood samples done by five laboratories in the Unites States, Canada, and Europe. They discovered up to 232 toxic chemicals in these ten blood samples. Nine out of the ten included the chemical BPA (hormone disrupting), and all ten samples contained chemicals used in can linings, flame retardant, synthetic fragrances, Teflon, food packing, computer keyboards, and much more. Nine out of the ten even included perchlorate, a solid rocket fuel component and potent thyroid toxin that can disrupt production of hormones essential for normal brain development (ewg.org).

More importantly... *these blood samples were taken from the <u>umbilical cord blood of ten babies</u>*. If this doesn't make us sit up and pay attention, I can't imagine what will. Obviously, these chemicals are permeating not just our own personal environment and bodies but unborn babies. And yet, the US government is still busy conducting studies or looking for proof that these chemicals are harmful or hormone disrupting. The European Union bans 1,328 chemicals, and the United States only prohibits eleven. In addition, the European Union requires the chemical industry to demonstrate that a chemical is safe in order for it to be used in products sold. In the United States, a chemical is presumed safe until proven dangerous. So until we see people literally having life-endangering reactions, you won't see it pulled from the market.

You would have to have enough of them not only have the reaction but also know enough to report it to the proper government authority (how many people would know to do that?) to prove the chemical is dangerous. Who is going to be reporting and compiling this data? Our government leaves it up to the chemical company to self-monitor and report. Do you think they will be in any hurry to do this? We can bet not....

This chemical onslaught creating xenoestrogens, disease, and cancers in our bodies has been increasing for decades as consumer demand for low-priced products has manufacturers using whatever is necessary to pump out the number of goods. Believe it or not, if our grandparents had a faulty toaster, they took it to be repaired. The same applied to almost any appliance or contraption they had. They did the same with shoes, boots, or jewelry. If it was broke, they fixed it. Manufacturers took the time to make high-quality items that would last longer. Today, I'm sure we can all agree we are a throwaway world. It's cheaper to buy a new toaster than it is to repair it. The same applies to almost every item we own. Therefore, manufacturers must continually deliver more and more items for us to consume.

Take a look at any dollar store or our big box retailer and you will see the true extent of our excessive consumption. Cheap, colorful products are loaded by the cartful by shoppers and taken home. We apparently are unaware of the toxic chemicals coating the outside as well as the interior in products such as jewelry, makeup, clothing, nail polish, beads, children's books and toys, and so much more. These are the same chemicals causing not only hormone disruption but childhood leukemia and other cancers. Unless we stop the excess consumption to fill our lives with more and more things, we will never see the chemicals reduced. It's the manufacturers job to stay in business. To do so, they must give us what we demand. When demand wants it cheap and in quantity, the manufacturer will use whatever they have to use to get the job done. Who has time for expensive, time-consuming studies on chemical safety? None of these companies are in business to take a loss. Paying for studies and tests would absolutely affect the bottom line, so don't look to the companies making these products to conduct studies and place package warnings voluntarily.

That leaves it up to us. It is literally up to each and every single one of us to look for quality over quantity. It just might cost more to buy a bamboo wood toy over a cheap plastic toy. It may mean Susie and Johnny gets two toys instead of fifteen on their next birthday. And that's the way it will have to be if we want to protect ourselves, our children, and our earth. This is much more than being a tree hugger. It's about our health and our children's health.

Additives to Avoid

Since we cannot possibly list all the things to avoid, let's look at some of the biggest culprits people are unaware are dangerous. Here is an extremely small list of some of the products that can contain a high level of chemicals. Honestly, I would be much ink and paper ahead to list things you can do to minimize your exposure (which I will do) rather than the immense number to avoid. However, I think it's vital we are aware of at least some of the more common, everyday products assumed safe that are culprits in hormone issues; these are slowly building in our children's bodies to emerge as hormone issues shortly into their puberty. And don't forget, puberty these days is beginning as early as eight years old. Start now with yourself and especially with your children. If you are blessed to have no issues at this point but you use the items listed below, it's just a matter of time. It's important for all of us to be aware of the products poisoning our bodies. We obviously cannot make changes if we are not made aware of the areas causing exposure. Let's take a look at the list of some of the most common culprits.

BPA

This is a chemical *known* to create synthetic estrogen or xenoestrogens. Here's the frustration of the slow-moving action of our government on chemicals known to cause disruption. BPA was actually identified in the 1930s for its synthetic estrogenic properties. And yet, it still on the market in today's products. According to the US Centers for Disease Control, at least 93 percent of Americans have significant levels of BPA in their bodies. Since it is a known estrogenic-causing material, it's high on the list of ones to avoid. Here are just a few products in which you will find BPA:

- Canned foods
- Plastic glasses
- Water bottles
- Dental sealants
- Coffee makers
- Water pipes

- Kitchen appliances such as Keurigs and K-cups
- Sodastream bottles
- Cash register receipts
- Paper currency
- Medical intravenous bags and tubing

Phthalates

Phthalates, pronounced Thah-lates, are made from petroleum used in many personal care products. They are used to soften and increase the flexibility of plastics. They are classified as endocrine-disrupting compounds (EDCs) and gender benders, according to CBS News' 2010 article "Phthalates, Are They Safe?" We find phthalates in a plethora of products. Remember our discussion earlier on how fragrances hang in the air and stick to our nasal membranes? Phthalates are one of the evil little compounds in fragrances that help them linger. Thus, almost any product with fragrance listed on the ingredients likely has phthalates. However, fragrance is far from the only culprit containing this chemical. Used in personal care products, phthalates improve texture, increase spreadability, and enhance absorption. Here are some products containing phthalates:

- Shampoo
- Cosmetics
- Lipstick
- Hairspray
- Nail polish and nail polish remover
- Toys
- Pacifiers
- Air fresheners

- Building materials (e.g., carpet, laminate flooring)
- Plastic dishes and utensils
- Clothing
- Cars (e.g., steering wheels, dashboard)

Avoid Plastic, Cardboard, and Styrofoam

The problem with BPA and phthalates is that they leak into whatever food or beverage you put in a plastic container, plastic-lined can, travel mugs, sippy cup, or plastic baby bottle (to name a few). If we put food or beverage in plastic and heat in the microwave, we are inviting chemicals. If you pour hot soup, leftovers, or drinks into plastic containers without letting them cool first, we invite them once again. According to Dr. Mercola's 2008 article "Don't Put Coffee in Plastic Cups," hot liquids in a plastic container or plastic-coated containers cause the chemicals to leak into the food or drink *fifty-five times* more rapidly than cold liquid. Now, if we take that plastic container, scoop in hot leftovers, or cover it with Saran Wrap or some other thin plastic covering while the food is hot...yikes! It's a chemical convention in the dish with your body ultimately becoming the host. When you clean up after dinner, let the food cool before putting it in containers

This same concept applies to putting plastic containers or utensils with plastic handles in your dishwasher. The extreme heat of the dishwasher is bound to release some of those chemicals to coat the other dishes in the dishwasher. This means not only the plastic dishes but likely all your dishes now have chemicals at the end of the cycle. Plastic never goes in my dishwasher. I don't use a microwave, but if I did, plastic with food or drink in it would most certainly not go in it either. A box of glass storage containers with lids is around $30 and goes a long way toward storage and is

215

surely a much cleaner option when it comes to chemicals leaking into your food.

Another area to be aware is hot coffee, cocoa, and tea from gas stations or restaurants. They are either lined cardboard (chemicals in the lining) or Styrofoam. Can you imagine the chemicals that would leak from Styrofoam when a hot liquid is poured into it? Obviously, if we pour something hot in a plastic container, there is going to be chemicals in whatever we put in it. One would think cardboard would be a much better option—and it likely is better than Styrofoam—but cardboard cups are lined with a type of plastic called polyethylene so the cup won't turn to mush. It does make it tough to swing by the convenience store and grab a cup of coffee, doesn't it? I make my own organic coffee at home and take it with me as much as possible. I also keep an empty ceramic mug in my car; anytime I am traveling and want a cup of coffee, I take the mug with me to the gas station or coffee shop and fill it. I've never been questioned on this, and apparently it's not all that unusual, as I've had some clerks mention they see this from other people as well. This usually ends up being one of those ten-minute conversations on chemicals in our environment with a complete stranger. (The more we share, the more we spread the word.)

One other concern on hot coffee and plastics is the popular Keurig coffee machine. Just imagine the number of chemicals in a cup of coffee made by steaming hot water running through a flimsy plastic pod to make coffee. It floors me that these are even legal. This includes the competitors that may have biodegradable pods. These would still have to have a lining containing constituents with chemicals to keep them from getting soggy as the hot steaming water runs through them. Where there are liners, there are chemicals.

Visiting your local health club or public park is a good example of how we need to become more aware of the infiltration of chemicals in our lives. There you will likely see people jogging, lifting weights, working, and sweating to be in good health and yet... what's often in their hands? In most cases, a plastic bottle of water or sports drink. Bottled water is a common and large source of chemicals for young females adding to their chemical buildup in the body.

Bottled water and sports drinks are the perfect example of how marketing has convinced us the contents of something is healthy when it's not. Most bottled water comes from a municipal supply system that is then put into plastic bottles. Even worse, most of these are soft plastic, which is higher on the chemicals list than the harder plastic. There may be times, such as traveling or a sporting event where plastic bottles of water are tough to avoid; drinking from the bottle is most often no healthier than the water fountain. Spring waters are better than the average bottled water as far as water choices. But it still comes in a plastic bottle. I've heard of people who buy all their drinking water in plastic bottles in an attempt to avoid the city water without realizing they have similar quality to the city water and likely worse due to the added chemicals from the plastic bottle. You will note some companies now advertise BPA-free on their bottles. However, the replacement chemical is often bisphenol-S (BPS) with another less known but equally toxic chemical called BPS. Not only does BPS appear to have similar hormone-mimicking characteristics to BPA, research also suggests it is actually significantly less biodegradable. Honestly, the safest bet is glass containers.

People also ask about the safety of metal water containers. I'm not wild about them, as I just don't care for the thought of any metals in my body. However, many health sites tout stainless steel as a safe alternative to plastic. It would be important to make sure it's all stainless steel; watch for little tricks to help lower the price such as aluminum or plastic liners and plastic caps.

It may be well worth it to invest in a reverse osmosis (RO) water system for your kitchen tap that removes fluoride, chlorine, and other metals and chemicals. However, with this type of system, be sure you supplement with a high-quality mineral supplement containing magnesium and trace minerals since the RO system will remove *all* minerals—the good minerals get removed with the bad stuff. I rent my system for $19 a month through Culligan. They change the filters once a year and do maintenance if necessary. To me, this beats buying and drinking from plastic bottles. Since I'm a big water drinker, I never leave the house without least one, if not several, glass water bottles filled with water so that I have my own water for the day rather than using the convenience store plastic bottles.

Fragrance

BPA and phthalates are only two of thousands of chemicals. While I cannot get into all of them in my limited space, I do want to cover one more dangerous additive in a tremendous number of our personal care products. We have covered it briefly, but let's expand upon it a tad more. Fragrance rates right up there with plastic as far as damage to the hormonal communication system and human body. Did you know that fragrance in your products can contain 120 individual chemicals, none of which have to be labeled? Ponder that number for just a moment. Chemicals. 120. That's up to 120 chemicals we willingly spray on our body, burn in the form of a candle in our home, plug into an outlet at the height of a little child's face, use on our clothes in the form of laundry detergent or fabric softener and hundreds if not thousands of other way we use them. A review of the scientific literature on female workers and breast cancer released by the Breast Cancer Fund in the 2015 article "The State of Evidence: Work Exposures and Breast Cancer" reveals hairdressers and cosmetologists have up to five times higher breast cancer risk. What do cosmetologists use on a daily basis? Fragrance- and chemical-laden shampoos, conditioners, gels, hairspray, nail polish/removers, and hair dye. Most of these are the very same products most other women (and children) use every day. They are just manifested in cosmetologists at an earlier age due to increased daily exposure. However, most women have that same exposure, but since it isn't as many times per day, it is just manifesting slower until our liver waves the white flag and we end up with a serious health condition. Cosmetologists are just representative of our entire population. They are the proof in the pudding regarding chemicals in personal care products and the dangers they invoke on our hormones and body. With the products used in a salon, we have not only the 120 potential chemicals from the fragrance but also the parabens. According to *Journal of Applied Toxicology*, these chemicals have been detected in breast cancer tissues at concentrations up to one million times higher than the estrogen (estradiol) levels naturally found in human breast tissue (2012). Let that information be your motivation to remove fragrance-laden personal care products from not only your life but your children's life. If you are a cosmetologist, consider doing as my stylist did. She has switched to working at a salon committed to safer, chemically reduced products.

Fortunately, more and more of us are becoming aware of the need for fewer chemicals. When you are shopping for safer products, it's important to read labels carefully. Manufacturers know many of us are looking for healthier, less toxic products. Therefore, the word "natural" is splashed across our personal care products as well as our foods. To be labeled organic does require following strict regulations. To use the word "natural" or "green" (in the case of cleaning or personal care products) on labeling in the United States, neither the FDA nor the USDA has rules or regulations. There is no standard for using these words. With the demand for clean or natural products booming, manufacturers are jumping on the bandwagon left and right to have the slickest, most colorful look possible on their products.

The fastest way of eliminating a product is to look at the ingredients. If I see the word fragrance in any way, shape, or form, it's back on the shelf (with a look of disgust on my face). This happens even with manufacturers who are stepping up their cleverness at labeling. Now they add "with essential oils" on the label knowing there are many of us who might like that option. When you look at ingredients from these products found at a retail store, I *still* see the word fragrance. If you have ever smelled a true essential oil, you know there would never be need for adding a fragrance smell or chemical.

Fluoride

While we are still on the topic of chemicals being introduced willingly into our bodies, let's talk briefly about fluoride. The one takeaway I'd like you to have on this topic is your right to refuse fluoride treatments at yours or your child's dental checkup. Refusing fluoride treatments has become a fairly common request, and I have yet to have my decision questioned by the various dental offices I have visited over the years. If you are pushed or questioned extensively, find a new dentist. This is your decision, and you are protecting yourself and your child. Fluoride is just one more example of the U.S. trying to treat an entire population without consent and also without extensive studies to prove its safety. It's added to our drinking water; it's in our mouthwash and toothpaste. It's applied at every dental checkup in our mouths where the highly absorbable membranes near our precious pituitary, amygdala, thyroid, and other hormone-controlling glands are located.

According to Dr. Grandjean and Dr. Landrigan, fluoride *is* a neurotoxin (*The Lancet Neurology,* volume 13, pages 330-338). The list of damage from fluoridation is lengthy, and the validity of its potential on tooth decay is shaky. If I were to take my chances on possible tooth decay from avoiding fluoride versus the proven damage from fluoride, tooth decay would certainly win. There is much we can do naturally to prevent tooth decay like avoiding sugar (big surprise), brushing after eating, coconut oil pulling (fabulous for tooth and gum health), and a clean diet. Removing fluoride from our brain and body is a much tougher proposition.

Don't *Give* it Up, *Switch* it Up

What's a person and especially young mothers to do? I won't lie; it ain't easy. Or at least it won't seem easy at first. After a little bit of practice, it gets much easier to play the "find the hidden chemicals" game. The personal care and food manufacturers are masters at this game, which makes it difficult when we go in search of a safe product. The good news is there is some help out there to up our game in response to the labeling tricks used by manufacturers. To help us in our search for safer products, there are several excellent resources. The website Environmental Working Group (EWG.org) rates products on a scale from 1 to 10 for toxicity. This is available for cosmetics, personal care products, cleaning products, and foods. In addition, there are at least two good phone apps you can use in the store by scanning the UPC code on a product. You will receive a rating as well as a list of what's bad in the product and other great info. EWG's app is called Healthy Living, and the other app is called Think Dirty, which isn't as suspicious as it may sound. Having these apps or others like them should make life easier when trying to figure out what's a clean product. These apps will help you in the search for what is safer.

The more you can make you own products, the better off you are. At least when you make it, you know what went into it. There are a multitude of recipes for cleaning and personal care products online using natural products such as baking soda, white vinegar, castile soap, essential oils, and coconut oil to name a few. I make my own sun lotion, pest spray, body lotion, hair conditioner, and cleaning supplies. Search Pinterest or Facebook for recipes or online for guides that have natural, homemade personal care and cleaning recipes.

If you're just not a DIY kind of person, the Internet has a plethora of reduced or zero-chemical products. Use the EWG.org website to research any product and, once you determine it's safe, use the Internet (Amazon Prime, anyone?) to get your product. I live in a rural area during the summer, and FedEx is a constant visitor due to my online ordering. Once you get used to your favorites and the supplier, it becomes much less time consuming. As you become accustomed to products that no longer have fragrance and the other added chemicals, you will likely have trouble even walking down the aisle of cleaning products or fragrance products at the store due to their powerful smell.

What to Avoid

Canned Foods

In the United States, over 85 percent of tin cans have a lining that contains BPAs—our estrogen-mimicking compound. This includes especially avoiding canned baby formulas but also all canned goods such as vegetables, beans, soda, fruits (especially acidic fruits), and tomato juice.

Plastics

As aforementioned, avoid them completely! Never heat food in plastic in the microwave. Avoid hot foods in plastic storage containers. Use glass containers for storage.

Food Dyes

When I see a child getting annihilated with sugar and food dyes in a picture from their birthday cake, I can't help but be concerned. If this was a rare occasion and children rarely got these things, that might be one thing, but our children get them on a daily basis with food like Jell-O, gummy bears, and birthday cake frosting modeled to look like the latest Disney character. To protect our children we need to be aware of our parties and daily reward systems.

Plastic Food Wraps

Plastic food wraps are thin, moldable plastics with dangerous chemicals that break down badly, particularly with hot liquids and foods.

Styrofoam or Lined Paper Cups

As we discussed, avoid disposable cups if at all possible. Make it a habit on any disposable cup—Styrofoam, plastic, or lined paper cups—to fill the cup at least twice with water and dump it out. This will at least help rid the initial accumulation of chemicals in the cup. Carry a glass bottle or coffee mug in your car so you can use these as your travel containers as much as possible.

Paints, Solvents, Lacquers

Observe the next time you go to a nail salon how the worker normally wears a mask to protect herself from the powder or chemicals. Truthfully, these masks provide minimal protection. But the other thought on this is where is *your* mask? Pay attention to the smell and the powder dust from the filing of the nails. Once I realized how many chemicals were in the air and going into my highly absorbable nasal membranes and breathed into my lungs, I gave up nail tips. I suggest, for the sake of your health, that you do the same and please, never go into these places while pregnant. Remember the umbilical cord blood study quoted earlier? That fetus is absorbing what we absorb.

Pesticides and Herbicides

Eat organic food as much as possible. If you don't buy organic, it's super important to be familiar with the dirty dozen list that you can find on EWG.org. These are the top 12 foods most likely to have chemical content. Soak your produce in a bowl of white vinegar with lemon for at least twenty minutes to try and help eliminate at least the exterior chemicals. This won't remove those housed in the food interior, but it's surely better than nothing.

Birth Control Pills and Spermicide

The chemicals in these synthetic hormones can literally reside in cell receptors for decades, long after we discontinue their use. BCPs are a creation made in a laboratory from synthetic chemicals and offered to unsuspecting women with zero explanation of the ramifications of their potential hazards. Spermicides inserted into the highly absorbable cell membranes contain chemicals and interfere with the vaginal bacteria balance leaving you susceptible to yeast and urinary tract infections.

Talc/Baby Powder

Often baby powder contains talc, which, when inhaled into lungs or absorbed through genitals into the body, can have cancer-causing effects. Along with the talc, many of these powders include other chemicals, especially fragrance (chemical public enemy #1 these days). It's an absolute no-no for babies (non-GMO corn starch of arrowroot powder is a nice alternative). Many young women sprinkle talc or baby powder in their underwear as a "smell fresh" habit. In theory, it's a good idea. In practice, the talc is exposing them to chemicals and hormone disruptors. There are lawsuits currently pending against Johnson & Johnson from young women getting uterine cancer at a young age due to using baby powder in their underwear without having any idea there were chemicals in the powder. Avoid these for you and especially for baby.

Household Detergents and Cleaners

If we listed the cleaners and detergents with chemicals, it would be a long, long list. Just know that almost every commercial cleaner on the market has chemicals in it. Be aware of allowing children to walk with bare feet or pets on floors that have been cleaned with chemical cleaners. If the label on the bottle makes it appear safe, take a peek at the ingredients and look for fragrance and other chemicals.

All Artificial Scents

Air fresheners are a big culprit in the high number of chemicals they emit. Room, car, and fabric fresheners, scented candles, and plug-ins contain fragrance. And remember, fragrance is made up of chemicals made in a lab. The sticky molecules absorb into the highly absorbable nasal membranes for disruption of hormone and health balance.

Fabric Softeners

This is a big one because we all think of cuddly little bear commercials or the snuggly soft feel of baby blankets. Instead of thinking of that warm fuzzy smell, think of those synthetic scents and toxins laying against your or your baby's skin and inhaled into what? Once again, highly absorbable nasal membranes.

Laundry Detergent

This is the same as the fabric softener or cleaners. Most laundry detergents include chemicals and scents.

Sunscreen

The chemicals in sunscreen go directly onto your and your child's skin. It is then warmed up on the skin, which opens the pores for better absorption. In addition, we have (what should be illegal) aerosol sunscreens. Chemicals in that sunscreen are now being absorbed through the skin *and* the nasal membranes. Living in Florida and seeing young parents, who undoubtedly love their kids, slather their children with sunscreen makes me concerned because they obviously don't know the number of chemicals in the sunscreen. It also makes me very angry because we know that they know when we think about the manufacturers of that product, yet they continue to advertise its use on babies/children and adults. We will discuss phone App's in our upcoming section on xenoestrogens. You can use one of these handy App's to help determine a safe sunscreen.

New Carpet and Furniture with Off-putting Fumes

If you have carpet installed or get new furniture, consider sleeping elsewhere for a few nights and leave a few windows cracked open, if possible. The fillings and fabric on furniture are loaded with chemicals. Fire retardants are another way we are preyed upon by the chemical industry in wanting to protect our family. The worst thing is that they don't even work. According to *Chicago Tribune's* Tribune Watchdog "Playing with Fire," "The average American baby is born with 10 fingers, 10 toes and the highest recorded levels of flame retardants among infants in the world. The toxic chemicals are present in nearly every home, packed into couches, chairs and many other products." As of 2015, it is no longer required to have these retardants "protecting us," but you will have to specifically ask and insist that your furniture, pillows, carpets, bedding don't have them. Although they are not cheap, one of the most important areas to consider buying organic would be your mattress. After all, we spend one-third of our life on our mattress.

Microwave

Do not stand near a microwave as it is running. There is no disagreement from the experts; they do emit radiation but there is the argument that it is supposedly safe as it's not DNA-altering radiation. We have seen study after study on different topics telling us how safe things are (e.g., birth control pills) to later find they have harmful effects. The microwave emits radiation. It is not difficult to move yourself and children away from it while it runs so please avoid it. Even better, consider ditching the microwave completely. While it may seem like we cannot do without it, I stopped using mine five years ago and was surprised how easily I adapted to the minute or two longer it took to heat something on the stovetop in a pan versus the microwave.

Teflon and Other Non-Stick Cookware

These are high in chemicals that leak into your foods. Titanium and cast iron are better alternatives.

X-rays

Avoid as much as possible. My dentist doesn't like that I don't allow X-rays, and I have had to switch from one who insisted I had to have a routine checkup with X-rays. If I have a tooth issue, I can't avoid the X-rays, but for both medical and dental, I do not seek out appointments for well care due to these types of invasive, unnecessary tests (in my opinion). It far too often turns into sick care.

Mammograms

Mammograms expose women to 1,000 times the radiation of a chest X-ray. Ladies, it makes no sense to radiate an area highly susceptible to cancer. This applies to mammograms as well as the subsequent tests involved if there are any suspicious areas detected such as MRIs and stereotactic biopsies. There is no question whatsoever that breast cancer is a huge concern. The number of young women (ages 25-39) in the United States being diagnosed with advanced breast cancer is increasing, according to the

228

2013 *Journal of the American Medical Association,* volume 309. Breast cancer *used* to be an older woman's disease but, unfortunately, not so much anymore. Rather than encouraging radiating the area as prevention, doctors should be advising on diet and toxin avoidance. However, as a reaction to the increasing numbers of breast cancer, we once again have a medical world encouraging early screening. This early screening involves mammograms that radiate breast tissue. The younger this begins, the worse the insult to the area and the higher risk it creates. Some great information that supports this topic comes from Dr. Mercola. He tells us,

> The primary hazard of mammography is ionizing radiation that may actually increase your cancer risk. According to a 2010 study, annual screening using digital or screen-film mammography on women aged 40–80 years is associated with an induced cancer incidence and fatal breast cancer rate of 20-25 cases per 100,000. This means annual mammograms cause 20-25 cases of fatal cancer for every 100,000 women getting the test. And now with the "new and improved" 3D TOMOSYNTHESIS mammogram, women will be exposed to even more radiation (mercola.com).

I am not saying we don't need caution but rather than routinely radiating this highly susceptible area, digital infrared thermal imaging (DITI) sometimes called thermography should be a highly considered alternative for women. The fact that it isn't is once again proof how important it is to be visiting health websites and reading natural health books to get alternative options to standard medical care suggestions. If we rely on the "experts" without looking at both sides of the coin, we are outsourcing our health to a profession, at this time, with some rather dismal statistics.

Vaccinations

A final note for this segment is regarding vaccines. Obviously, this is a hot topic and highly debated. There's a saying, "every anti-vax parent was pro-vax until their child had a vaccine reaction." This was the case in our family. We were absolutely for vaccines and thought those who didn't believe in them must be wrong. After standing in the ER watching our daughter in seizures the very day she received her Gardasil vaccine, our minds were certainly awakened to the possibility we might need to rethink our stance. We had initially done a quick questioning of the gynecologist who recommended the vaccine and were assured it was safe. She told us her two teenage daughters were getting it as well. Obviously, if a doctor would use it with her children, I assumed it must be safe and did zero research. I won't go into further discussion other than to encourage you to research this area. Again, read articles not only from the standard medical websites but also the natural health websites to get more balanced input. We get one tiny body to protect. It's worth spending some time looking at both sides of the discussion on this hot topic.

Reducing Toxin Exposure

What are things we can *do* to reduce toxins exposure?

- Look for non-toxic paints. There are companies that make much safer interior paints than the standard commercial paint. These safer formulas can be formaldehyde free, emit minimal VOCs, and they also can contain sealing properties that reduce outgassing.

- Wash your hands after handling anything plastic, cash register receipts, or packaging. Treat plastic just like you do after handling something you think might have germs; wash your hands.

- Wash all children's (and your) clothes prior to wearing them. Fire retardant chemicals and dyes on our clothes (and furniture) is a big source of chemicals.

- Look for glass baby bottles. There are many online sites as well as big box stores that carry glass bottles with rubber-coated linings.

- Look for glass dishes, and ditch any plastic dishes.

- Purchase glass storage dishes over cheaper, thin plastic containers.

- Bookmark websites that have safer products and articles on reducing chemicals so you can easily locate them when you need information.

- Make or purchase chemical-free personal care and cleaning products.

- Always type in the words "organic" or "chemical free" when searching for products online. Amazon sells many organic products and is one of my favorite sites for variety and speed of delivery. I also love the many customer reviews for discussion on whether the product is truly chemical free. The Internet is a fabulous resource for locating chemical-free products from water bottles to baby pacifiers, toys, and sippy cups.

Chapter Fifteen: Xenoestrogens

Even though we have several chapters on hormone balance, We can sum up the top root cause contributors for most female hormone imbalance issues with three main areas: diet, chemicals, and stress. These are our main contributors to hormone imbalance. I want you to keep these main contributors always at the forefront of your mind. When you keep these as your main focus, it will prevent you from getting distracted if and when you have extensive blood work done and get your results showing areas out of range. While I am by no means saying there is no need for blood tests, I will say they can send you chasing down a road to taking a boatload of supplements or meds for that particular condition, which can distract from *why* you have that particular situation. It's good to know what is out of range, but remember it may once again be the smoke detector—not the cause of the fire.

We have touched upon this earlier so I shall not dwell, but for now, always keep in mind the need to zero in on the interaction of the entire body and the initial, potential disruptors for that interaction. For example, when you focus on clean diet and lifestyle, you impact liver health. This can clear the body or out-of-range thyroid hormones may eventually become a non-issue (or at least less of an issue). Any or all of the following relate to the basics and ultimately impact our hormone balance. For instance:

- When we limit our exposure to high amounts of chemicals, grains, and sugar, our liver stress (where estrogen is synthesized and metabolized) may be eased and excess estrogen levels may drop.

- When we reduce sugar or gluten, the inflammation contributing to extreme cramping may ease.

- When we limit sugar intake, the liver has the potential to rest and regenerate to ease ovarian cysts, PCOS, and other female conditions.

The body corrects when we give it a fair chance by stopping the disruption. If we try to correct one area by supplementing with birth control pills or progesterone without reducing the chemicals, diet, or stress issues, we are treating the area that needs support but not removing the reason the area needs that support. The focus must be to find and reduce the core disruptors. Otherwise, the progesterone supplement you use to help with estrogen dominance likely will require a higher and higher dose over time or become ineffective with your hormone balance going right back to estrogen dominance. Let's expand on the overall picture.

1. We inhale, ingest, and absorb a shocking amount of chemicals from our personal care products and food.

2. The body's clearing house, our liver, cannot clear out all these chemicals so it directs them to be stored in our fat cells to protect us.

3. Chemicals continue to get piled on our body (through our daily use of personal-care, cleaning, and food products). The stored chemicals remain and do not get released from the fat cells to be excreted. These fat cells, designed to protect us from the overabundance of chemicals, begin to secrete powerful estrogen mimickers called xenoestrogens (pronounced zeno-estrogen).

4. These powerful xenoestrogens with poor liver health contribute to estrogen dominance and progesterone deficiency, a major cause of

many female hormone-related conditions including hormone-related cancers.

5. Our liver cannot keep up with the continual bombardment of chemicals and sugar. It waves a white flag and gives up or at least greatly reduces its job of clearing our bodies of dangerous substances.

6. When the liver—the clearing-house of chemicals and excess hormones—becomes compromised or overloaded, we start backing up all these excess chemicals and hormones. It tries to deal with this excess in any way it can. One way is to continue to direct them to our fat cells. If we don't have enough fat cells for storage, the body will create more fat cells to accommodate the storage of these toxic and dangerous chemicals and hormones.

7. The body has a greatly compromised clearing-house (Liver), so now it does whatever it can to try and rid itself of these excess hormones and xenoestrogens. This will manifest in a variety of ways. It can come in the form of severe cramping, continual bleeding, several periods per month, fibroids, female cancers, as well as any other condition created from a stressed, chemical-laden body on overload.

Estrogen dominance contributes to low levels (almost nonexistent in some women) of progesterone, our estrogen balancer. Progesterone is our calming hormone (mood issues), our relaxation hormone (cramping), and our hormone that causes uterine lining to thicken to prepare for egg implantation (fertility).

An Unwelcomed Guest

Normal female cycles and reproduction involve a fine balance *of all* hormones. When we have a powerful intruder (xenoestrogens) caused by chemicals creating these powerful estrogen "mimickers", that balance is greatly disrupted. This applies to younger women's conditions as well as older ladies and also men. None of us is excluded from their powerful effects to disrupt our hormones. Let's look at this unwelcome, dominant estrogen in the following scenario.

Let's say you are estrogen. You and a couple of your girlfriends, progesterone and testosterone, get together for a glass of wine at the local restaurant. You are all looking forward to some girl time to chat and relax. As estrogen, you are the most feminine of the group; you like your lipstick and high heels. Progesterone is the calming influence for you other ladies; she is the calmest, most relaxed lady in the group. Testosterone is a tad more aggressive and athletic than the rest but knows her place and is a supportive friend. You are all enjoying your time together with each contributing equally for a balanced conversation. Suddenly, you look up to see your neighbor xenoestrogen (pronounced zeno-estrogen)—we will call her Xeno—has decided to stop in unannounced and join your group. None of you want or need her to join your group, but you are not given a choice as she heads right on over to your table to be included. She takes a seat (invasive xenoestrogens don't wait for an invitation, they move right on in) and orders herself a cocktail (chemicals from everyday products). Even though she is unwelcome, she jumps right in talking about her busy day, her annoying husband, health issues, blah, blah, blah. Each of you prefers she leaves so you do your best to ignore her. However, she is a very pushy lady and won't back off. Even worse, the more cocktails (chemicals) she consumes, the louder she becomes.

Your group can find no good way to eliminate (excrete) her unwelcome company. One by one, each of your group stops contributing to the conversation (reduced hormone levels). Progesterone becomes the quietest and the first to drop out due to her calm, gentle personality. Eventually, the rest of you (estrogen and testosterone) reduce your contribution to the conversation as well (reduced hormone level) and drop out of the conversation. Xeno is fine with this because she loves being the center of attention. She's the strongest personality and takes over to completely dominate the group (body). The relaxed group contributing equally (balanced hormones) is no longer balanced. It's become one person—hormone—who disrupts and dominates everything. You eventually threw in the towel and gave up trying (reduced or extremely low-level progesterone, testosterone, and good estrogen in blood or saliva testing) to bring back group balance because it's impossible to compete with her continual and increasing noise. Meanwhile, Xeno is happy. As long as the chemical cocktails continue, she plans on staying.

A Never-Ending Cycle

How the heck did this happen and who invited Xeno anyway? Actually, *you* invited her, and you continue to invite her every single day. You love your makeup and ice cream. You love chips, crackers, hairspray, fabric softener, and pretty smelling candles. We are females and doggone it, we are not giving up our makeup, hair gel, perfume, or room freshener. Thus, we invite xenoestrogens into our lives. We invite them in a variety of chemicals that convert in our body to an invasive, dominant, disrupting force.

When we are younger, we don't know Xeno exists. When she first visits, your body is pretty good at handling her. This is mainly due to your built-in exterminator of the chemicals, your liver. Over time (it could be years even decades), your liver gets overwhelmed and gradually filters out less and less of this powerful estrogen mimicker. As the liver starts getting overworked and overwhelmed, xenoestrogens create chaos in not only hormone balance but the entire body.

Eventually, we go to the doctor who says nothing about chemicals and xenoestrogens. Actually, most times, your doctor is unaware of chemicals as the cause of Xeno and her bad behavior. Instead, he/she focuses on your blood test results and medications. What likely happens next is tests (if they were run) will show hormones out of range and very likely your doctor will prescribe birth control pills since this is the current "first line of defense" for women's hormone imbalance. Your doctor also normally advises using some pain medications from the drugstore to get you through the rough days. Xeno is delighted at this little turn of events because, first, the doctor ignored her supplier (chemically laden personal care products and food) so her odds of hanging out in your body just increased exponentially. Second, the chance of the liver clearing her out just reduced greatly due to the addition of synthetic medications that adds to the burden on your Liver. Xeno's dominance results in progesterone getting her feelings hurt (levels out of range) and refusing to join in the girls' club anymore because she is overwhelmed. Even though progesterone is not participating much anymore, the continual onslaught of chemicals and meds gives Xeno new girlfriends. The new girls aren't gentle like progesterone. They are xenoestrogens—just like Xeno—who are dominant and strong.

As time goes on, you are frustrated you aren't feeling any better plus you're now gaining weight. You are getting a tad more desperate to feel more like your old self. You go back to the doctor and possibly have more tests run to try to figure out what's going on in your body. Xeno and I can surely tell you what's going on, but remember, nobody is considering a high sugar diet, chemicals and xenoestrogens a cause for your issues.... You are given a few more medications plus refills on original medications. Out the door you go happy that all will be well soon. Xeno is happy, too. She now has her girls' club growing daily. Each application of makeup, each dose of medication, each inhalation of fragrance (in the form of room freshener, sunscreen, perfume, hairspray, candles), each processed food with preservatives and sugar brings her more members to help bully or kick out the other members of your girls' club—*normal* estrogen, testosterone, progesterone, along with the other steroid hormones that they disrupt and overwhelm.

Unfortunately, this cycle of meds and unwelcome side effects will continue as long as you are unaware and/or unwilling to ditch the things you love—the food and products introduced when you were a child and that have been used day after day, week after week, year after year. This also means Xeno likely has a very powerful girls' club already organized in your body.

The above scenario leaves out a whole range of other body reactions that would be happening during this time. But, for our discussion and analogy, we remain focused on the steroid and sex hormones. This analogy is also a simplistic view of why hormone-level testing could possibly be misleading. If progesterone is the first one to give up, your tests will obviously show low progesterone. Therefore, supplemental progesterone may be prescribed. Certainly knowing your levels and using the progesterone gives us a start and hopefully relief, but remember, progesterone is quiet (low) due to the dominance of Xeno caused from chemicals. We will get into why and what kind of progesterone, but for now, consider that the issue obviously isn't progesterone itself. There is a reason progesterone (or any other hormone tested) is low or out of range. If you only supplement progesterone without looking for the root cause, the load on the liver is added due to the progesterone supplementation as well as chemicals and food toxins continuing their onslaught. Progesterone (bioidentical) supplementation can offer great relief which is good—but we need to remove the cause of the low progesterone-chemical sugar and stress disruption.

In one aspect, body fat is our friend. The liver is performing exactly as it should in an attempt to protect us by directing excess hormones (created by chemicals, sugar, grains, and medications) away from your vital organs to fat tissue to be stored until at some time the body can deal with disposing of them. The bad news is that fat cells eventually excrete xenoestrogens as a result of the chemical confusion within the cell and as an attempt to deal with the chemicals. Therefore, even if you carry excess body fat, our chemical exposure can be so high that the body creates more fat as your "sewage disposal" site to store these chemicals. Unfortunately, it's a double-edged sword because the more fat you carry, the more estrogen you produce and vice versa.

We live in an estrogenic, overly feminized fish bowl. Men are every bit as affected as women. Chemicals and toxins men ingest, inhale, and apply to their bodies make our males powerfully disrupted as well. Remember the opening of our discussion of hormone balance with the foreign country planning to take over the by interfering with both male and female hormone balance? It's not too far-fetched, is it?

Saying Goodbye to Xenoestrogens

The great news is removing chemicals and eating a healthy diet can help the body do amazing things to reach homeostasis. The other great news is the liver is the one organ in the body that can regenerate. But these things happen only if the body is given the opportunity to do so. This is where we all have our own personal responsibility for our health. Who is going to rid that annoying, disrupting Xeno from your body? The beauty of this is how unbelievably simple it is to make a difference in what she is doing to your body. There is also beauty in finding how much power you hold versus relying on a third party to fix things. The only one who can get rid of Xeno is *you*. Show her and her friends the door by eliminating chemicals and sugars. We get no "get out of jail free" card. No pill, no oil, no vitamin, no supplement, and no surgery will remove her and allow your body to start healing. Chemicals and poor diet contribute to the root cause of why we are seeing this epidemic of hormone-related conditions, and they're also the reason no medication on earth will fix the problem. The only way to heal is to offer toxin-free food and products that go on and in our body.

You may choose to look the other way, but you can never say again that you did not know. Reducing chemicals, a healthy diet, and working to correct past damage is our prescription and one that stands a tremendously higher chance of correcting hormone-related health issues.

As a quick review, why do we become estrogen dominant? Here are some main causes:

- Eating a diet high in processed foods, which are a source of added sugars and chemicals in the form of preservatives, stabilizers, thickening agents, and dyes, equate to chemical interference in the body.

- Personal care products that include makeup, air fresheners, body lotion, shampoo, conditioner, body wash, fabric softener, etc. These contain powerful xenoestrogen-creating compounds.

- Chronic stress, which interferes with restorative sleep, places strain on the adrenals and the thyroid glands; this increases cortisol production. Elevated cortisol can block pregnenolone receptors, which can interfere with our progesterone production (one cause of low-progesterone levels).

- As we approach perimenopause, our estrogen/progesterone levels fluctuate tremendously with both estrogen and progesterone beginning their initial decline. Often progesterone declines at a much faster rate leaving many women suffering from estrogen dominance.

- The pituitary gland is a gland highly susceptible to damage. A damaged pituitary will result (among many interactions involved) of pituitary deficiency will affect estrogen/progesterone levels.

- Conventionally grown foods where standard practice is to use large amounts of pesticides and fertilizers. Our meats and dairy products (especially milk) contain hormones and antibiotics administered to our animals

- Prescription medications that can interfere with liver function (where our estrogen is processed) include pain meds, synthetic hormones, such as the birth control pill, synthetic progesterone, testosterone, and estrogen as hormone replacement therapy (HRT).

- Leaky gut or other gut issues, which can affect the liver thereby interfering with our chemical/toxin filter process. This ultimately places excess physical stress on the body, which raises cortisol to interfere with estrogen-detoxification processes in the liver and block progesterone receptors.

We are now done with this section on the power of chemicals to create xenoestrogens that greatly disrupt our endocrine system and hormone balance. From here we move on to one powerful way to get relief for many of the female conditions we see today—supplemental progesterone.

ESSENTIAL GUT & HORMONE WELLNESS

Chapter Sixteen: The Positives of Progesterone and Pregnenolone

Progesterone is our calming hormone. Progesterone protects against the undesirable effects of unopposed estrogen. Progesterone is important to central nervous system functions. Dr. John Lee, M.D. and author of the book *The Breakthrough Book on Natural Hormone Balance* states, "Progesterone is concentrated in brain cells to levels twenty times higher than that of blood serum levels." Is it any wonder then, when women's progesterone levels take a big spike during pregnancy and then drop suddenly after birth and delivery that postpartum depression can be caused by a progesterone deficiency? Or is it any wonder that an inordinate number of women are struggling with mental health problems such as anxiety and depression? Balanced levels of progesterone contribute to better sex drive, bone health, skin appearance, mental health...the list goes on. The list of unopposed estrogen conditions is below, and it is an extensive list.

I return to the one question that frustrates more than one female: *Why* do we not know more about this helpful hormone? Why does our doctor not know more about it? One reason is that natural/bioidentical progesterone cannot be patented by a drug company. Thus, there is no value to teaching its benefits to your doctor, my doctor, even the specialist at the most highly touted medical clinic. If you wait for and rely on the advice you get from someone who has been highly influenced by an industry that has no desire for you to learn of natural/bioidentical progesterone, you may be headed down the road of unnecessary suffering, as we did. Our point in this book is to introduce you to the subject. Hopefully, you will continue learning by expanding your learning after the information here. I guarantee it will be time well spent.

Before I begin, I want to make clear that the progesterone we will be discussing here is actually progesterone *supplementation* or adding progesterone to the body. For a body low in progesterone, *adding* it can be a breath of fresh air with wonderful relief to some of the symptoms caused by estrogen dominance. If you are *not* struggling with female hormone-related issues, you may want to consider *support* of progesterone already at healthy levels with an essential oil or supplement. Oils or supplements are created to support the human body. They are not designed to deliver at a strength level that will add; rather, the low amounts offered to the body will help support the endocrine system and body. This along with proper diet, chemical removal, and supplemental support may help the body do its job maintaining homeostasis and negate the need for supplemental levels. But, if you exhibit hormone-related health issues such as those listed below, you may want to add via the delivery forms listed below.

While adding progesterone is not the ultimate answer for the root cause of many of our female hormone-related issues, it can be amazingly effective for our symptoms. Before you ever, ever consider a surgery or harsh injection treatments, I would strongly encourage you to give added natural/bioidentical progesterone a try for relief. Then focus on making diet, chemical removal, liver support and stress changes as possibilities to hopefully help resolve the issue of why you have low progesterone. The goal is to eventually come to balance through these things and taper off the bioidentical progesterone as you incorporate changes to naturally balance progesterone. In the meantime, supplementation can be helpful with low risk of side effects.

Adding progesterone can raise progesterone levels to give relief but over time can place stress on the liver (remember how vital it is to hormone balance to maintain proper liver function?) and other organs. It has potential for relief but the question remains. *Why* do we have the symptoms that demonstrate a need for the added progesterone? It's vital to find the reason behind your body's low progesterone production. And in almost every case, it is environment, diet, and lifestyle. Therefore, we cannot assume we can just use added progesterone and our problems are solved. They likely will feel that way since you get relief, but long term, the need to remove chemicals, clean up diet, and remove stress remains.

Let's review some of the conditions that are a result of estrogen dominance/progesterone deficiency:

- Miscarriage
- Fibroids
- Infertility
- Early onset puberty
- Cramping
- Excessive bleeding
- Migraines
- Postpartum depression
- MS
- High blood pressure
- Fibrocystic breasts
- Low sex drive
- Excess estrogen promotes blood clotting (a side effect listed with birth control pills) thus increasing risk of stroke

- Anxiety
- Depression
- Osteoporosis
- PCOS
- PMS
- Hot flashes
- Menopause issues

Considering this extensive list, is it not beyond a little bit frustrating that progesterone does not come up in conversations at the doctor's office? At the risk of redundancy but with the hope of emphasizing, I repeat that natural progesterone was never offered to Karly in spite of fifteen years of appointments with some of the best gynecologists, surgeons, and specialists the state of Minnesota had to offer including Mayo clinic. Yet an MD natural health doctor informed us in one hour-long seminar of the answer to helping the symptoms as well as what is the cause of her situation (xenoestrogens). If your blood tests show low progesterone levels, you should request a prescription for a supplemental bioidentical progesterone but it's important to know what form is safest with least interference to the body. Therefore, consider the following:

Synthetic Hormone versus Bioidentical Hormone

Prescribed synthetic progesterone with progestin is greatly different than a natural/bioidentical progesterone prescription. Even worse, because many doctors are unfamiliar with natural/bioidentical progesterone, they will either try to prescribe you the synthetic we just discussed, refuse to give you anything, tell you there is no difference, or tell you it won't help your condition. If you are given a prescription by your doctor, a synthetic hormone is the most common type prescribed. It is a hormone made in a pharmaceutical laboratory from synthetic (man-made) chemical compounds with potential risks greater than any benefit. Because they are synthetic, they cannot act in the body like a natural source and are not a good choice.

I would encourage you to look for a doctor more familiar with bioidentical/natural hormones. These are synthesized in a laboratory from plant sources. Hence, the term natural or bioidentical versus synthetic. The doctors familiar with this form are usually doctors who specialize in bioidentical hormones and the type of doctor I would look for if you seek relief through progesterone.

The significant difference between synthetic hormones and bioidentical hormones, however, is how they act in the human body. Synthetic hormones like Premarin, a synthetic estrogen, and Prempro or Prometrium, synthetic progesterones, have a molecular bond that is not recognized by the human body. Therefore, they are not metabolized efficiently and have undesired side effects. Conversely, the body recognizes bioidentical hormones because their molecular structure is like that of the hormones produced naturally. Because the molecular structure of bioidentical hormones is more recognized by the human body, they are more efficiently metabolized and have not been shown to increase carcinogens in the process.

There are a variety of delivery forms for adding natural/bioidentical progesterone, and it can be obtained at a higher dose level through your doctor (as we've discussed) or it can be purchased online or in some stores as a progesterone cream—at a lesser strength than that from your doctor—to be applied topically.

Different Forms of Progesterone Delivery

Synthetic Progesterone Capsules

Synthetic progesterone is in capsule delivery form. As already mentioned, I would not recommend this form, as there are too many potential side effects. This is usually the form of delivery most conventional doctors prefer. It most likely is not natural progesterone, but I am listing it here to make you familiar with it.

Capsule or Wafer/Troche/Tablet Bioidentical/Natural Form

These are the forms often used by a health professional that specializes in women's hormones. It also is the form most likely used by functional medicine or naturopath doctors. Capsule is one common form of delivery and is the form some doctors prefer. One thought on this delivery form is that it must run through the digestive system and liver; a fair amount is not utilized well so bigger amounts have to be used to get the desired effect. The other option would be what we call sublingual bioidentical progesterone that comes in the form of troches/wafers or a tablet. They are placed under the tongue or between cheek and gum to dissolve and be absorbed into the bloodstream. This is the form of natural progesterone delivery used by Karly with great effectiveness. Since it is absorbed directly to the bloodstream rather than swallowed, it bypasses the liver and kidneys and enters the bloodstream directly. The advantage on the capsule or troche/wafer/tablet form is that the bioidentical progesterone comes from a natural plant source.

Creams and Gels

Creams and gels normally contain the desired bioidentical form of progesterone and can be prescribed at a higher strength by your doctor and are applied to the skin directly. They can also be purchased online without a prescription at a lesser strength. If you or your loved one does not have severe symptoms, the non-prescription cream/gel form of delivery may be preferred since it would support but wouldn't be adding as high an amount as the prescription cream or the capsule/troche/water delivery form. Due to the lower amount of natural progesterone levels in almost all non-prescription creams, it may or may not be strong enough for those with severe symptoms.

If you have severe symptoms, I would start with the cream but, if symptoms continue, I would encourage you to visit with your doctor to look into getting troches/wafers/tablets. However, if your symptoms are not severe, the cream/gel option may be effective and may decrease the chance of delivering more than is necessary. Try the lower amount offered by using a cream/gel, beginning with the recommended amount for at least a week or two and if you don't see improvement, I might increase the amount used. If that eventually does not do the job, then look into finding a doctor who will work with you to obtain the bioidentical troche/wafer or capsule form of delivery. If what you are using is not working, use more and more often at least until you feel better and then slowly back off on the amount unless symptoms return. Try to find the balance of not overusing but getting enough to help the body. You can find creams/gels online or in health stores. I would look for one that delivers at least twenty mg of natural progesterone per dose. The following are a couple of good ones recommended by those who used them with beneficial results:

- Emerita ProGest Cream can be found on Amazon and comes in a lotion/cream. It contains no petroleum or mineral oils, and it is paraben free and fragrance free.

- NatPro Organic comes from soy, but it is processed to extract the progesterone with no estrogen-like effects common from soy products.

- AllVia Progensa 20 from Integrated Pharmaceuticals comes in a pump container dispensing the progesterone in a cream form and can be found on Amazon.

Where some issues come into play with adding progesterone is that many women use too little, and it irritates cell receptors to increase their symptoms. I compare using too little progesterone to tickling or irritating the cell receptors. When we offer enough, the cell receptors (and symptoms) should be saying, "Thank you very much!" If they aren't, it's either not enough progesterone or perhaps you need a different form of delivery.

Regardless of the reason, if you have estrogen-dominant symptoms, natural/bioidentical progesterone is one of the safest, most effective constituents you could offer your body. The amount of progesterone to use is not dependent on your weight, size, height, or age but on your symptoms. The number of various instructions from different sources, the varying creams and potencies, the concern over how to use it and the misinformation has caused many hundreds of women to abandon using it assuming it does not work—and that is a downright shame. Work on the hormone balance checklist as well as stay in touch with your health professional and your odds of success for your particular issue will have much better odds.

Birth Control

We can't move forward until we discuss the risks and ramifications of birth control pills (BCP). This is one of the first methods of handling female hormones doctors will use when a woman struggles. Karly was prescribed these at fourteen years old as a potential help to her endometriosis symptoms. Now knowing the risks and long-term ramifications of synthetic hormones, you can bet we would have walked out of the doctor's office at that time. But we didn't know. Let's look at the statistics of number of women using these damaging, synthetic hormones in birth control pills:

- BCP are used by 28% of women in their reproductive years.
- Some 762,000 women who use the pill (9% of all pill users) have never had sex and use the method almost exclusively for non-contraceptive reasons.
- Four of every five sexually experienced women have used the pill.
- The birth control pill is the method most widely used by white women, women in their teens and twenties, never-married and cohabiting women, childless women, and college graduates.

Many birth control pills contain *high levels of estrogen*. At the very least, they contain synthetic, powerful estrogen. Considering we've had a lengthy discussion on the contribution of xenoestrogens to our hormone balance, this should be an immediate red flag. BCPs convince your pituitary gland that you are pregnant and don't need to ovulate. How did the medical world ever decide this was not a monstrous effect on hormone balance with eventual ramifications to the one using the pill? This would explain the extensive list of potential side effects of these drugs.

Anything synthetic is much more difficult for our liver to process or

251

for the body to excrete. This means, even after you have discontinued using the pill, the constituents from the synthetic form may hang out in your cell receptors for years. It doesn't matter what brand, what type, or what assurances you get that a particular pill is safer. The fact is every single prescription birth control pill on the market has some form of synthetic hormones. And a synthetic hormone is a recipe for hormone balance interference. For now, be aware synthetic estrogen and progestins, such as that in birth control pills, contributes to depression, gut health imbalance, increased cancer risk, candida along with a long list of other potential side effects. As one example of how important it is to stay informed, if you have depression and you are on the pill, rather than take you off the pill to see if you improve, you will likely be prescribed an anti-depressant. Do you see why that might be a backward approach to a hormone imbalance that affects mood?

Infertility

Along this line of synthetic hormones, there should be a discussion on infertility and fertility drugs. Some 7.3 million Americans, or 12 percent of the population in their reproductive years, are infertile, according to the Centers for Disease Control and Prevention (CDC). This is a staggering statistic, and one that leads us back to our discussion of chemicals, stress, and diet affecting a woman's fertility. You or your doctor may believe your situation and problem are unique and the only way to get pregnant is with dangerous fertility drugs. However, I would implore you to clean up your environment and diet to see what changes might happen before ever submitting to these drugs that can and will have long-term side effects including increased cancer risk.

I currently have three out of three friends who have uterine cancer; they had fertility meds 15-20 years ago. We can say the meds have improved and are safer, but in my eye, this would be hogwash. Powerful levels of synthetic hormones—no matter the form of delivery—are worrisome. Does my heart break for any female struggling to have a baby? Yes, it surely does. But filling a body with chemical hormones is not the answer. Look to the source of infertility. There are many potential possibilities from high sugar intake, high stress, overweight, past birth control pills use, and estrogen dominance/progesterone deficiency to name a few. Also, consider the male may be affected by estrogen dominance and exposure to years of chemicals in food and personal care products. This can result in hormone balance including low testosterone for him just as much as the female can be affected. The same efforts to help his levels would apply—diet, chemicals, and stress. (Don't forget diet includes sugar!)

Look to the hormone balance checklist and make every effort to abide by it if you really want a healthy baby and momma. If all else fails, read and research carefully before deciding whether to undergo fertility treatments. The very last thing you should do at this emotional time of your life is make quick, rash decisions or rely on a medical person who only knows one way to ramp up your fertility—synthetic hormones.

Why You Need Extra Progesterone

It may seem hard to believe that one thing, natural progesterone, could make a difference in the many female health issues listed earlier. After all, why would something as simple as natural progesterone ever be able to help with severe bleeding, cramping, depression, miscarriages, fibroids, infertility, osteoporosis, and hot flashes?

The big problem I will emphasize here is *there is* a reason our daughter and all women with severe hormone-related issues need to supplement with natural progesterone. Women who need and benefit from natural progesterone are almost always estrogen dominant (as we have discussed earlier in this chapter). The ultimate end result of estrogen dominance can result in many of the female conditions we have listed. Remember progesterone hormone is calming and soothes; estrogen will aggravate or escalate the situation (especially powerful xenoestrogens). But also remember supplementation of progesterone should be a temporary fix while you work to remove the source of the xenoestrogens.

Pregnenolone

Many women have been able to successfully balance hormones without the use of either bioidentical progesterone or pregnenolone (our next topic). Some have great results with cleaning up diet and environment along with using a high-quality organic maca root powder (from the radish family) or Chaste Tree Vitex capsules to help with estrogen dominance. Younger through post-menopause aged women alike can try these as well as certain foods, such as flax seed or flax oil, dried dates or prunes, green peas, and alfalfa sprouts (avoid unfermented soy). These are only a few supporting foods and supplements for estrogen balance. We just spent a significant amount of time on natural/bioidentical progesterone, and I am going to spend a bit more time discussing bioidentical pregnenolone.

The Precursor for the Curse

If we look at the health conditions from disrupted hormone balance, it's apparent this is the curse of modern society. So let's take a look at something coincidentally labeled a precursor to our steroid hormones—pregnenolone. Pregnenolone is often referred to as the mother hormone. The next precursor in line is DHEA. Both pregnenolone and DHEA are not actual hormones but precursors to your steroid hormones, and are synthesized from cholesterol in the liver. Pregnenolone and DHEA are upstream of hormone production. It can be utilized by the body to support *any deficient hormone area.* This is pretty darn amazing! Pregnenolone can be synthesized in a way to help support the lacking hormone. Cholesterol is the raw material from which pregnenolone is produced, then DHEA and eventually all steroid hormones. We will discuss how highly important cholesterol is in your diet later, but keep in mind it is vital for proper hormone synthesizing processes.

How do we know where to focus first in this merry-go-round cycle of hormones? This is where having a precursor like pregnenolone can be helpful. As a precursor to your hormones, it has the substance that carries the ingredients necessary for synthesizing and supporting a hormone wanting support. If we are lacking progesterone, pregnenolone can be converted to progesterone more heavily than estrogen and vice versa.

In the article "Common Hormonal Problems in CFD, Dr. Sarah Myhill writes, "Starting off with pregnenolone means that all steroid hormones can be naturally synthesised in the correct physiological balance" (http://drmyhill.co.uk/). When viewed from the natural process in the creation and utilization of hormones in the body, the use of bioidentical pregnenolone may be a good starting point. This applies to men as much as women. Starting further up the chain of reactions by using bioidentical pregnenolone can be much less disruptive than trying to supplement individual hormones. Personally, if I struggled with one of the estrogen-dominant conditions (see our earlier list), I would start with the hormone balance checklist as well as bioidentical pregnenolone and/or progesterone as potential relief for my symptoms. With this, you could eventually taper off the progesterone and later the pregnenolone as long as you also:

- Reduce chemicals in personal care and cleaning products
- Reduce sugars and carbs in your diet
- Reduce stress

You should also be sure to include cholesterol foods in your diet to support production of pregnenolone and progesterone hormones. The ideal situation is to find a good doctor well versed in these areas. You may need to highlight and circle some of this information and the importance of this natural hormone chain of events so that you can ask him/her to discuss them with you and, hopefully, prescribe them (only bioidentical/natural, of course).

If you try bioidentical progesterone and get limited results, it may be well worth trying pregnenolone to possibly boost its production and effects. If your doctor is familiar with bioidentical pregnenolone, it's likely in the capsule form. However, I would push for the sublingual troche for increased absorbency and avoiding the liver's first pass effect that the capsule— bioidentical—form will follow. However, the capsule might do it for you if your doctor is set on it; something is likely better than nothing. Just be sure you don't accept synthetic progestins. Remember, if the prescription doesn't come from an apothecary/compounding pharmacy, it is synthetic.

Pregnenolone is formed mainly in the adrenals. Once again, we are back to the emphasis of avoiding stress due to the impact it will have on our adrenals-where our cortisol (stress hormone) is synthesized, interfering with proper amounts of pregnenolone production. Its possible symptoms can get worse before they improve. As the progesterone, pregnenolone, or other bioidenticals start to take effect, it's likely the bad estrogen gets its walking papers from the cell receptors. This is a good thing and should eventually ease.

It's important to note that bioidenticals or any hormone-related product will likely interfere with birth control. Therefore, if you use these, you will need to consider alternate methods of birth control than the pill. (This is a good idea anyway considering the damage they do to your body.) The alternatives to birth control pills aren't easy or perfect, but it's important to research and choose the best alternative for you and your partner.

To educate your partner on the risks to you for birth control pills, pull out the sheet of side effects that come with the prescription or have him consider that in 2002, a well-documented study of post menopause women and hormone-replacement therapy was halted because women taking these synthetic hormones showed such a high risk of breast cancer, stroke, heart attack, and blood clots that continuing with the study would have been unethical. What do we use that contains the same type of synthetic hormones (estrogen and progestins) used in this highly dangerous study? Birth control pills. Freely prescribed and recommended to our unknowing and trusting young women on a daily basis across the country. Inform your partner of these very real facts and side effects. If you want, as additional support, show him the statistics for female-related hormone conditions listed at the beginning of the hormones' section; one of the solutions listed often in this book (and many health articles on the Internet) is to avoid synthetic hormones, which is exactly what birth control pills are—synthetic and risky.

It may appear, with all this discussion on prescriptions for bioidentical hormones, that I am pro meds. Nothing could be further from the truth. However, if you have severe symptoms from one of the typical hormone-related conditions, it may be necessary to use some of the above suggestions. Using these bioidentical prescriptions is at least using natural components and is surely safer than prescription synthetic hormones. I continue to emphasize the importance of gut health, diet, chemical removal, liver health, exercise, and stress relief to eventually get away from needing to add hormones—even bioidentical hormones. However, it can take as long as a year (or more) to get resupplied and rebalanced. So be patient and have your doctor occasionally run tests levels to see if you can decrease your supplementation. When you start feeling better, take time to support healthy levels then slowly taper after a period of giving your body some relief. Never discontinue suddenly (this applies to all medications). If younger ladies eat well and take the necessary actions we have discussed to support their hormones, supplementation should not be necessary *after* getting back in line. Post-menopausal women will have a reduced level naturally and can consider if they want to support with bioidenticals or stick to using foods/supplements that can support healthy hormone levels.

Progesterone as an estrogen balancer and relaxing hormone can be helpful. But it's not the end result answer. Clean up products and diet and reduce stress as a good place to begin. Get your progesterone in line with added progesterone or pregnenolone if necessary and then slowly reduce it as you get the toxins/stress out of your life.

Hormone balance is attainable. Once you achieve it, you will be amazed how much better your energy and emotions are. To achieve this balance will involve a change in mindset. You must have a strong conviction to avoid prescription medications, fragrances and chemicals, and finally, a conviction to believe what is on the end of your fork *is* the most powerful medicine available.

Chapter Seventeen: Liver Care

If there is one area that likely gets overlooked in the balance of female hormones, it's the liver. And yet...this is one very important organ that deserves great respect *and* great care. What? Liver care doesn't sound exciting? Actually, the more you take a look at the ingenious design and many functions of our liver, the more you come to realize what a highly important unsung hero it is. At the very least, it should be interesting to know that, by caring for it, you generate support in working toward hormone balance. Let's take a good look at a few of the functions of the liver. This is important stuff! Our liver:

- Secretes bile, which aids in digestion. Remember the vital importance of absorbing our nutrients!

- Produces and utilizes cholesterol to manufacture pregnenolone—our precursor to the all-important progesterone needed as a balance to estrogen.

- Breaks down excess estrogen and chemicals into a more excretable form to eliminate from the body. We want Xeno and her friends gone from our body, and the liver is just the guy for the job!

In addition to making and utilizing cholesterol for our master hormone and mother hormone synthesizer, the liver *is* your chemical filtration plant. It filters chemicals, but it also helps clear excess estrogen. The liver converts excess estrogen by converting it to a form more easily excreted by the body.

The problem is the poor treatment and burden put on our liver with the sheer volume of chemicals and xenoestrogens being put in and on the body.

Intrinsic and amazing as it is, the genetic design of the human body passed down to us from our forefathers never included how to clear fragrance, parabens, glyphosate (in pesticides/herbicides), phthalates, triclosan, or the *thousands* of other chemicals linked to hormonal imbalance, toxicities, reproductive health problems, and even cancer. These things did not exist even one hundred years ago. How could our liver, developed from ancestors that had clean living, possibly keep up with clearing this many chemicals? The sad fact is it can't. While our poor liver is working overtime to try and clear the overload of chemicals already in the body, more are being added each day from our fragrance-laden shampoos, conditioners, body washes, lotions, makeup, hair sprays, and perfumes—and that's just to start the day!

If a body part could cry out for help, I suspect our liver would be the first to do so. Actually, in its own way, the liver is crying out for help in the form of manifesting female hormone-related symptoms. In addition, the liver is so overworked trying to clear the body of these chemicals, it can't possibly keep up with its regular job of synthesizing cholesterol to produce the necessary master (insulin) hormone and mother (pregnenolone) precursor hormone (called pregnenolone steal) that ultimately affect the cascade of hormones further down the chain of estrogen, testosterone, progesterone, etc.

Liver Attack

Our environment is laden with chemicals. To add insult to injury, what comes along to hamper liver function *even* further? Sugar, grains, pasta, bread—these and any other forms of food we ingest in today's diet that break down to sugar in the body. The bad news? Sugar annihilates liver health. (Have you noticed there really isn't one single, good thing about sugar?) Let's look at the trifecta of liver attack:

- Birth control pills, pain-relief meds (including over-the-counter acetaminophen, aspirin, and ibuprofen), narcotics
- Excess sugar and grains in almost every diet today
- Chemicals (plastics, fragrances, insecticides, fertilizers, etc.) in our personal care and food products

This really is only a partial list of what the liver must deal with, but it gives us an idea of the amount of work our liver needs to do on a daily basis. It's amazing our liver even gets us to adulthood considering how much it is forced to endure from today's environment.

Here's the real kicker on the fallacy of testing in this area. Liver abnormalities in your lab work often do not appear at the onset of the problems but after years of suffering from a sluggish liver. While we tend to think elevated enzymes means upcoming potential damage, they really mean damage is done. It is not a yellow light or warning. It means danger. After fifteen years of birth control pills, repeated (almost continual) doses of narcotics, depression meds, and untold amounts of Tylenol and Advil, Karly had her liver enzymes tested at my request. Her enzymes were slightly elevated so her doctor told her to avoid alcohol for a week or two. Are you *kidding* me? This is literally the type of care we are dealing with. If those liver enzymes are elevated, it is a liver literally screaming for help; it's drowning in a sea of narcotics and pills. Since her condition was a female hormone condition (endometriosis) that had estrogen fueling the fire and since the liver is responsible for breaking down excess estrogen, she badly needed a healthy liver—the same as each and every female on this planet.

If we wait until enzymes are elevated, we have a big job of mopping up the damage. That's assuming our liver hasn't given up. In that case, you have bigger problems than hormone issues. Thankfully, the liver is the one organ that can regenerate, which is possibly a big reason Karly is still with us today. Any other organ would be permanently damaged. However, she paid the price in hormone imbalance (particularly estrogen dominance) from the liver being unable to do its job. I suspect her liver began getting overloaded at a young age by drinking three glasses of milk every day and having one or two plug-in air fresheners to make her bedroom smell nice. She also started using makeup at a very young age (as did her friends in school) and, of course, from the time she was a baby, we used milk in plastic baby bottles, fragrance-laden shampoos, conditioners, and body wash. Is it any wonder she had hormone issues from her very first menstrual period? Fifty lashes for her mother for missing the boat on toxins avoidance! Our next big mistake was following standard medical protocol of birth control pills. Looking back, I understand completely why she didn't stand a chance of getting better and why things continued to escalate.

Another female might say she uses all these things and doesn't have endometriosis or hormone issues. Remember, health issues will manifest in the most susceptible part of the body. Perhaps for them, it's the thyroid, allergies, asthma, ear or sinus infections, or if they are really lucky, they don't have any health issues...yet. However, if the onslaught continues, the liver will eventually give up or at least greatly reduce its efficiency and the inevitable issues will surface. We were unfortunate (or maybe fortunate since it taught us so much) the issues started at a young age. Sadly, there are far too many for whom it starts young: for the ladies starting puberty at eight years old, it starts young. For the adolescent girls with depression, it starts young. For the young boys with undescended testicles or a deformed sex organ causing urination problems, it starts young. For the twenty-seven-year-old young lady with uterine cancer, it started young. The list goes on of young people affected by an overload of xenoestrogens from chemicals and sugar that the liver cannot clear. I implore you to do all you can to remove the damaging factors so that you and your young ones do not join the growing list of statistics.

MTHFR

One of the genes involved to help the liver is known as MTHFR. A naturopath or functional medicine doctor may test for a MTHFR defect. This is one of these areas that may be helpful, but I caution, once again, not to get so hung up on dealing with it that we believe we are defective and there is nothing we can do. Never forget our big influence on our liver. When we help the body realign and balance through good diet and chemical and stress removal, it can do an amazing job of overcoming many defects. While this may not be true in every situation, it can be beneficial in many cases. Therefore, start with the Focus Four of gut health and the hormone balance checklist. If you don't get relief after a few months of applying these principles, you can always begin testing for defects. But first and foremost, start with helping the body achieve balance by easing the stressors and toxin load and providing nutrients through a healthy diet.

Caring for Our Liver

What can we do to help our liver so that it can help us have hormone balance? First and foremost, avoid chemically laden products and sugar.

Avoid excess alcohol and diet sodas or sports drinks. Then, offer that hard-working liver some support.

The following is a partial list of things to use for Liver support.

FOOD	SUPPLEMENT
• Celery Seed	• Glutathione
• Lemon in Water	• High-quality B vitamins (especially B12)
• Apple Cider Vinegar	• Avoid antacids, which block B12 and nutrient absorption
• Pure Water	• Vitamin C
• Cholesterol-rich foods (Eggs, butter, ghee, fish)	• Milk Thistle
• Grapefruit, Walnuts, Garlic, Turmeric	• SAMe (Methionine)
• Cruciferous foods	• Dandelion Root
• Broccoli, Cauliflower, Cabbage, Brussels Sprouts	• Turmeric (in addition to whole-food Turmeric)

Note cholesterol-rich food on this list. We certainly want cholesterol in our diets. Pregnenolone (mother precursor hormone) and insulin (master hormone) are produced from cholesterol with cholesterol produced in the liver. Once again, if the master and mother hormone are not supported through cholesterol as part of good liver health, how can we expect the other hormones further down the line to function properly? Thus, *low* cholesterol (contrary to popular belief) is *not* necessarily a good thing. Low cholesterol may be caused by many factors including an overload of toxins in the liver, causing poor production of cholesterol or poor diet with little to no cholesterol due to modern diets of processed foods. Low cholesterol also can be due to marketing and doctors convincing us to avoid cholesterol (butter, fish oil, eggs) or induced by cholesterol-lowering drugs.

Ironically, if you visit many of the top medical health websites, they still list cholesterol as a bad thing and even list margarine (no, no, and _no_) as a healthy alternative. Add healthy fats containing cholesterol to our diet (which gives us approximately 25 percent of cholesterol) and let's care for our liver to get our approximate 75 percent from our liver cholesterol.

This discussion on the liver is super important for healthy hormone balance, but it is also vital to whole body health. Therefore, I'm going to repeat the summary of three areas our liver contributes to health and hormones:

- Secretes bile, which aids in digestion. Remember how vitally important it is to digest our food to absorb nutrients!
- Aids in manufacturing progesterone and pregnenolone. Remember these are the good guys needed as a balance to excess estrogen.
- Breaks down xenoestrogen (the bad girl) and chemicals into a more excretable form so we can eliminate them from the body.

I mention the liver breaks down xenoestrogens. I should actually say the liver _tries_ to break down as many xenoestrogens as it can. The liver is designed to break down and excrete excess estrogen produced naturally by the human body, not _xeno_estrogens. The powerful, unnatural xenoestrogens are tremendously more difficult to break down than our natural estrogen. Not only is the liver working overtime and at full pace trying to break down the bad stuff, we are continually adding more through processed foods and personal care/cleaning products.

Everything we breathe, ingest, or absorb through the skin gets into the bloodstream and eventually passes through the liver. Because the liver is the body's primary detoxifier, it supports healthy hormone production and is a link to our digestive system. Keeping it healthy is critical to your overall health. This organ is the unsung hero of the major body organs, so love your liver!

Chapter Eighteen: Reducing/Alleviating Stress and Emotions

"Every emotion, every thought is associated with a biochemical reaction in your body." —Christiane Northrup, MD

The next step on the hormone balance checklist is reducing stress and emotions. A belief held by natural health practitioners is at least 70 percent of physical health issues are associated with emotional health issues. This makes total sense when you really think about it. Think how your shoulders tense, jaw clenches, stomach hurts, and heart rate increases when you are upset or unhappy. When emotions are not in harmony, circulation in the body is hampered. Without proper blood flow, every single body cell, tissue, organ, gland, joint, and system has impeded blood flow for it to operate properly. We are all well aware of the need for circulation to an injured area for proper healing. The same concept applies to the importance of circulation on a day-to-day basis for the entire body to operate properly. The body-mind connection is a vital component—rather it is the *main* component—for good health.

The human body has an amazing capacity to protect us. We have discussed how toxins entering the physical body are filtered and excess is stored in fat tissues until a time we clean up our act enough to deal with them. If we continue to pile on toxins, we never eliminate the stored toxins. Eventually, they manifest into a health condition in the weakest and most susceptible body part.

Negative emotions and stress are toxins to the mental state of the body and are handled in a very similar way as physical toxins. In its wisdom of trying to protect us, the body will store harbored emotions in a body part that can best handle it (often the liver). Eventually, if we don't deal with the emotion, the stored anger, resentment, hurt, or fear overloads the system. It will manifest in the part of the body most susceptible at the time.

Dealing with unwanted emotions is a concept some people have difficulty accepting. They are quite sure they have dealt with past issues, they believe they are tough and don't need to, or they assume it will eventually just go away on its own. However, when we hold in emotions—no matter how tough or resilient we think we might be—they will eventually emerge in the form of a health issue. Therefore, we want to cover what creates stress, why it can be harmful, and ways to release it so that we retain or regain good health.

We never realize how tense we are until we relax the body.

We never know how much we need to relax until we realize how tense we are.

This is the conundrum of the root of many health issues. Needing to be aware of a problem so that you can remedy the problem *yet* not knowing you even have a problem. Becoming aware of whether your jaw is clenched, your shoulders are tensed, your eyes are narrowed, or your neck is tight is the first step in realizing there is a problem. Once we are aware, we can start to focus on learning to relax or let go. Once we relax, we realize how tense we have been, and how much it has been affecting us.

Most of us are well aware we should avoid stress, and most also believe we have it under control. Therefore, we are quite sure we do not need to be concerned with articles or chapters pertaining to stress and its impact on our health. I bet if I were to really dig deep on the emotional health of a roomful

269

of women, at least 40-50 percent would have hormone balance or health affected by stress in one form or another. Actually, depending on your definition of stress, that number could jump to 90-95 percent. So just in case, let's have you read through this next section, OK?

The Effects of Stress

Stress comes in many forms. Every *single* person—thus, their body and mind—is under stress to some degree. What is stress? It isn't always the obvious high-stress matters of marital issues or death in the family. It can be the common, everyday issues that slowly become unrelenting such as waking every night with a baby for more than the normal time of a few months. It can be a job that requires more work than you can get done each day. It can be a mother-in-law often stopping by with unwanted advice. It can be the effects of a surgery. It can be a teenager (that's stress all by itself for sure!) in the household. It can be thousands of small things that accumulate over time. We all have some form or forms of stressors. We may not be able to physically remove the stressors or emotional issues from our life, but we can learn how to react to them to a certain degree. As a matter of fact, we *must* learn how to react. Study after study will concur, uncontrolled stress—be it rushed lifestyle, financial issues, marital problems, or pent-up emotions of hurt, anger, resentment, and fear—will affect our health.

Dr. Hans Selye was a Canadian endocrinologist who spent several years studying the effects of chronic stress. He showed that if you stressed rats, their adrenal glands enlarged to produce more stress hormones (cortisol and DHEA) to allow them to cope with that stress. If the rat had a break and a rest, the adrenal gland would return to its normal size and recover. However, if the rat was stressed without a break, he would be all right for some time but then suddenly collapse and die. When Selye looked at the adrenal glands, they were shriveled up. The glands had become exhausted.

In other words, our body unquestionably reacts to stress but has its limits. What it can't handle is continual, relenting stress and harbored emotions that cause stress to the nervous system. It can't handle stress that disrupts our sleep long enough that we can't seem to return to normal sleep patterns. The rejuvenating, rebuilding, regenerating effects of healing in the body come during sleep. If we don't have normal sleep patterns, health issues will eventually emerge and bite us in the hind end. That's an absolute health fact.

If for no other reason than hormone balance, it is well worth learning about relaxation and stress-reduction techniques. Harbored emotions or daily issues cause stress, which greatly affects hormone balance. Chronic stress induces high cortisol, which puts stress on our adrenal glands and reduces thyroid function, progesterone, and pregnenolone production. Remember that progesterone is our feel-good hormone and balance to estrogen; it is a major player as our calming hormone as well as an influence in a tremendous number of female functions such as cramping, bleeding, infertility, miscarriages, fibroids, and depression/anxiety.

Stress also increases heart rate and interferes with sleep. This increases cortisol levels, which affects mental health and ultimately does what? It increases stress. Whew! What a vicious cycle! All the pills, all the treatments, all the best supplements in the world cannot and will not cure a body under stress if we don't remove its source. As an example of this, remember my friend Kristine with postpartum depression? Her excellent bioidentical hormone doctor had her using both pregnenolone (based on an article I sent with her to her appointment) and progesterone. She also prescribed a small amount of bioidentical DHEA based on her blood tests. Her doctor, rightly so, felt this should bring Kristine relief quickly.

For years, Kristine's diet has been healthy organic, non-GMO, and vegetable rich. She avoids the standard estrogenic fragrance-laden products. Between her bioidenticals and her lifestyle, she should have seen relief quickly. But she didn't. This was a puzzler since it appeared we had all the components in place to help her on her way to recovery. But, for some reason, she wasn't making progress toward improving. There seemed to be no reason she shouldn't improve. That is until we started looking at the stress part of this equation. Kristine readily admits she had poor adrenal health prior to getting pregnant. She had an extremely high-pressure job, and she'd been doing intense cardio workout sessions three times per week for over a year. This was apparently raising her cortisol and placing stress on the adrenals (where progesterone is made) prior to getting pregnant. Her job along with extreme workouts and a poor diet at the time due to a rushed, high-stress lifestyle took its toll on her. She first had her aforementioned miscarriage and then, without waiting for at least six months to let her body recover, she got pregnant again. This time, her body produced a beautiful baby, but she paid the price as her body expressed its exhaustion and hormone imbalance by manifesting as postpartum depression. Let's take a look at what likely is going on for Kristine:

- High-stress job and intensity exercise leads to chronically stressed adrenals and poor thyroid function.
- Miscarriage possibly occurred due to adrenal stress, which causes progesterone insufficiency and difficulty holding a pregnancy.

- Pregnancy without full recovery means more demands on the already stressed adrenals, causing adrenal exhaustion and continued progesterone deficiency.

- Birth of baby and disrupted sleep to care for baby for a full year causes the adrenals to be highly affected, resulting in continual impact on progesterone production.

- Stressed adrenals and the resulting progesterone issues equate to postpartum depression.

- Kristine struggles with postpartum depression. Baby wakes often during the night the first year of life, causing interference of Kristine's sleep patterns.

- Poor sleep increases stress, which increases cortisol.

- Chronically high cortisol continues to interfere with pregnenolone and progesterone production even with the bioidenticals involved.

- High cortisol interferes with sleep, resulting in a cycle of poor sleep/high cortisol.

Remember that progesterone is our feel-good hormone, and progesterone levels are greatly related to depression. My heart goes out to Kristine whenever I talk to her or see her. It's evident she is exhausted and greatly struggling. The long and the short of it is that Kristine will need to find some stress-reduction methods (and probably need help with the baby for a while) to lower her cortisol if she is ever going to get some restful sleep to help break the high cortisol-production cycle and rest her severely stressed adrenal glands. Remember the study at the beginning of this section on rats with severely stressed adrenal glands? The result of continual stress is a very real and dangerous health issue. Until the stress is managed, the progesterone/pregnenolone combo can only have limited effect. This reinforces when we say we must deal with root cause to help our supplementation be effective.

Why did Kristine struggle so badly with birth and delivery and baby's first year of life when other women don't? While not everyone struggles with postpartum issues, there most surely are other women who do. The number of women with postpartum depression is escalating much like other female health concerns have been escalating. The question remains, why do these women struggle with postpartum depression when you or I might not? My guess, with studies to support this theory, is for most of these women, there is a severe hormone imbalance and/or chronic stress prior to getting pregnant. The body will always steal from the mother before the baby. So, we get a healthy (or relatively healthy) baby. Once that baby is delivered, however, the imbalances that have been building are finally expressed, causing adrenal exhaustion, postpartum depression, irregular periods, or some other physical/mental issue.

Kristine's issue was her job, past health issues, and intense physical workouts raising her cortisol. However, take the steps listed above as she descended into poor health and plug in whatever your stressor might be. For many, the numerous chemicals and/or birth control pills affecting their hormone balance might be what tips them over the edge.

For other women, it may not be a high-stress job and extreme exercise that cause the issue. It may be makeup, personal care product chemicals, a poor diet, recent surgery or illness; it may be financial, marital, or other emotional issues. It may be a combo of any or all of these things. The underlying basic triggers remain (e.g., chemicals, diet, stress) with the results manifesting differently in each person. Whatever your stressors might be, be aware hormone imbalance does not happen overnight. It has been building for years (much like cancer does) before making its appearance.

The current and accepted lifestyle in today's modern world is for people to continue to push themselves. Many cope with a great deal of stress. It often happens during this time that we enter stage II of adrenal fatigue where we are pumping out extra adrenaline. Most women actually feel pretty good and energetic in this phase. However, if we were to get a picture of their adrenals, it's very likely their adrenal glands are swollen or enlarged because they are working overtime to pump out the adrenaline required to keep going. Depending on diet, exercise, and toxin exposure, a person can last with stage II adrenals for years or even decades. But everybody has their breaking point. And that breaking point will emerge as a major health issue.

If the body becomes stressed or if it has buried emotions, then stress cortisol interferes with proper digestion as well as the proper production of adrenal hormones of progesterone, estrogen, cortisol etc. Our adrenal glands get busy pumping out the undesired cortisol while detracting them away from the building, regenerating, and balancing hormones needed for normal hormone function. This is our pregnenolone steal that ends up interfering with our all-important hormone, progesterone, that we badly need to help deal with the overload of xenoestrogens and to maintain proper hormone balance.

We are all susceptible to the highly damaging effects of cortisol. Therefore, it's important women—and especially young mothers raising their children—evaluate and learn the importance of saying no. Do the children really need gymnastics, hockey, soccer, basketball, or whatever the current activity might be? Yes, it's important to give them opportunities, but if these opportunities keep you running 3-5 nights per week after working all day, it may be time to pick and choose. They will survive but you will feel the effect if you don't.

We heal or maintain balance when we use positive methods to deal with our everyday stressors or buried emotions. Positive thoughts encourage energy flow throughout the body to aid with regenerative sleep. The following suggestioins are part of the basic recipe to help Kristine's body, my body, or your body heal itself. Obviously, we must include the basics of healthy eating and toxin removal. However, if we don't learn to recognize and react to stress appropriately, none of the other steps matter. Supplements, healthy food, bioidenticals, nothing can balance if we don't recognize and work on how we react to our stressors. Whether you do or do not think you feel stressed or have buried emotions, I suggest you try some of the techniques we will discuss in this next section on stress. It's bound to feel good regardless of what you might think about your stress levels.

How to Deal with Stress

I won't dwell on some of the standard methods used to relieve stress or let go of stored emotions other than to give them a quick mention. Some of the standard methods include chiropractic care, acupuncture, massage, and other natural methods. There is great benefit in these but it's also good to incorporate methods you can use at home on a daily basis. I will spend a little time on my favorite methods that can be done in short time periods each day.

The 4-7-8 (Relaxing Breath) Exercise

One of the biggest helps (at least for me) is a proven stress reliever involving your breathing. The majority of us tend to be shallow breathers. We get busy or involved in our work, and the last thing we think about is our breathing. Breathing deeply is not only great for relaxing, but it's also the primary way of moving the fluid of our lymph system. This method is much more than just taking a deep breath occasionally. It's a structure breathing exercise used often in yoga or meditation and made known to many of us by Dr. Andrew Weil. I use this breathing method almost every night as my "sleeping pill" once I turn out the lights. I also use it occasionally during the day if I catch myself tensing my shoulders or feel my heart rate going. You can use this breathing while at work, driving, standing in line, or most anywhere.

One important thing when you first begin is to have your back straight so you can feel proper breathing flow. Since deep breathing can cause some people to get a tad lightheaded, Dr. Weil recommends starting with only one or two breaths at first. This breathing exercise is often used in yoga or meditation. There are many videos demonstrating it by Dr. Weil available on his website, **www.drweil.com**. The following is his explanation of how to incorporate this breathing:

For this method, place the tip of your tongue against the ridge of tissue just behind your upper front teeth, and keep it there through the entire exercise. You will be exhaling through your mouth around your tongue; try pursing your lips slightly if this seems awkward.

- Exhale completely through your mouth, making a whoosh sound.
- Close your mouth and inhale quietly through your nose to a mental count of four.
- Hold your breath for a count of seven.

- Exhale completely through your mouth, making a whoosh sound to a count of eight. (The video I saw on this had instructions to say the word "ha" as you exhaled with a big final "ha" on the eight).

- This is one breath. Now inhale again and repeat the cycle three more times for a total of four breaths.

Always inhale quietly through your nose and exhale audibly through your mouth. The tip of your tongue stays in position the whole time. Don't do this breathing exercise while driving or in public until you're sure you won't get lightheaded. If you feel a little lightheaded when you first breathe this way, it will pass. I combine this breathing exercise with a few essential oils for full benefit from the technique. See the section on essential oils if you are interested in more information.

Let it Go

A suggestion for dealing with negative thoughts that keep invading your head at bedtime may seem like an obvious one and yet, far too often, we are guilty of not doing it. The suggestion is to stop chewing on what is bothering us, or as Elsa from *Frozen* tells us, "Let it go." My mother used to tell me, "Give it its five minutes and be done with it for the day." I believe she was on to a good concept. It's one I use often and would recommend to you as well. If you wake during the night and start stewing on an argument or upcoming work or whatever the sleep-disrupting issue might be, give it five minutes of worrying and thinking about it, then force your thoughts away. I guarantee it will try to reemerge a few times but push it away and change your thoughts; incorporate the 4-7-8 breathing technique so you are distracted with counting breaths and can drift back off to sleep.

Positive Thoughts

Along the line of dealing with stress for healing, we also want to learn the power of positive emotions. Positive affirmations help us with how we speak to ourselves. Self-speak is not a "woo-woo" thing. Self-speak is powerful to the emotions, to an uplifting lifestyle, and to the body's healing process. Literally, where your mind goes, energy flows. If your thoughts are focused on health issues or the wrong someone committed against you, your nervous system energy and circulation slows. Your body will tighten and get stuck in that gear. We cannot expect to improve because circulation and energy are impeded. When you think positive thoughts and speak to yourself with positive affirmations, such as "I will heal. I will take charge. I can do this," the brain, energy, frequency, and circulation will flow to this area of the body.

This may seem as though it won't have much effect if you are just venturing into the whole body (holistic) way of thought, but remember we discussed that up to 70 percent of physical issues can be related to emotions. Consider how many times we read an article on a cancer patient miraculously being healed by a positive mindset. Obviously, he/she had to juice vegetables, eat healthy, and remove toxins as well. However, in almost all of the cases you read, they claim their biggest change, as part of the healing process, was their attitude. They made their mindset "I will heal," and they practiced easing the mind to take stress off the body. They included positive thoughts and affirmations, which literally increase positive energy flow throughout the body.

How do we become happier? It takes conscious thought and practice to change the habit of being negative. No one wants to be negative.

279

We slowly slide into that habit *or* we've had some very negative things happen to us. Either way, if we continue in a negative vein, whoever or whatever caused us to first go down the negative path will continue to have influence over us until death. Make a conscious effort to catch yourself anytime you find yourself being negative; turn your thought patterns into a different pattern of optimism and positivity. We literally open new receptors in the brain when we do this. It brings more blood flow throughout the body since it eases tension. Register for emails to websites that make you feel good, or read some good books that are uplifting, funny, and encouraging. Friends or associates you surround yourself with will have a huge impact on your mental thoughts and attitude. Choose wisely. You do *not* have to be afraid you are rude if you choose not to allow a negative person into your life. Kick out the bad, and bring in the good in your relationships and in your mind.

EFT-Emotional Freedom Technique

Another favorite practice I have used that makes a powerful impact is a method called EFT. This one takes a little more learning but is not super difficult. Dr. Mercola says,

> EFT is a form of psychological acupressure, based on the same energy meridians used in traditional acupuncture to treat physical and emotional ailments for over five thousand years, but without the invasiveness of needles. Instead, simple tapping with the fingertips is used to input kinetic energy onto specific meridians on the head and chest while you think about your specific problem—whether it is a traumatic event, an addiction, pain, etc.— and voice positive affirmations (mercola.com).

Visit the website of Dr. Mercola at mercola.com and search EFT to find specifics on how to practice this method. I vouch for the effectiveness and how easy it is to use.

Yoga

Yoga has been used for thousands of years to great effect. The gentle stretches, breathing, and strength training of the individual muscles are greatly therapeutic to the mind and body. There is a multitude of different methods. Some have somewhat complicated names such as Hatha, Vinyasa, Kundalini, Bikram, and more. My recommendation is to start with a beginner's course (if you are not currently practicing yoga). Start with the basics, get comfortable, and, just like any exercise, keep it simple so you don't quit. There are hundreds of videos on YouTube or elsewhere that you can use to learn about yoga. There are a number of great DVDs that you can use at home. I personally don't use a structured yoga program. I end my simple sessions of hand weights with stretching legs and back muscles. This works for me, but there are many people who love and practice yoga daily with great results for stress reduction.

Meditation

A sad loss in our lives today is the loss of the state of stillness, especially in our world of overstimulation from cell phones, computers, emails, errands, kids, and all the other busyness of life. How often does a person just stop, enjoy quiet time, and breathe? Far too seldom. I believe it's one reason we have difficulty dealing with many of these topics under this section on stress. We aren't used to stopping, breathing, and just being. Honestly, if you are a young mother, just going to the bathroom without an audience is difficult.

How are you supposed to find time to breathe and meditate? You may have to go sit outside in the car while hubby keeps the kids busy to deep breathe, use EFT or meditate after the kids are in bed. Work to set time aside to shut down the brain activity for a while, during the day but especially at bedtime. If we don't slow down the brain activity prior to bedtime, it keeps going while we sleep and we lose a good portion of the regenerative actions we so badly need. This is the entire purpose of meditation—calming the brain to benefit the physical body. Meditation involves deep breathing (great for lymph and nervous system), focusing on stillness, and taking time to shut down. There are well-documented studies on its benefit and, again, you can start with some simple videos or books. Keep it simple so you keep at it.

Prayer

Growing up Catholic (at least in our local church), I never really learned to sit down with a Bible and study it. I didn't feel as though we prayed as much as we recited and repeated. Therefore, I wasn't comfortable with praying or talking with God, which meant I didn't have a relationship with Him. We all have our breaking point. When unrelenting stress continues, something has eventually got to give. The body will compensate and continue to move forward sometimes weeks, years, or even decades depending on your health when you enter the period of stress.

When life knocks you on your knees, you are in a perfect position to pray. During our worst years where we literally thought we would lose our daughter to the narcotics and injections, my health declined enough where life did "knock me on my knees." I found great solace in prayer and developed a relationship with God. If this is not where you are in life or you are unwilling to seek that relationship, you can move on to the next section.

But for those who want a relationship but don't know how to pray, I hear ya. I found the best process was to just begin—just talk to God out loud like a good friend (which He is). This is the first step in prayer. We just talk. We say our thoughts and our wants out loud. As my friend George says, "We can't assume He knows. If we can't spend the time to literally ask for what we want, God can't know our wants and that our heart is open to a relationship." So I talked and constantly asked that He keep my daughter alive and, if it was part of His plan, to reduce her pain. My prayers were "I know you can't heal her Lord; she's too sick. But I pray you reduce her pain so this beautiful young girl doesn't have to suffer so badly." Miraculously, not only did her pain get better, He led me to the knowledge we needed to heal her. By doing so, He gave me the information to try to help others in a similar situation of getting no answers from modern medicine and being left without hope. I have found great comfort in prayer over many instances in the ensuing years.

If you are at a point you would like to build a relationship with God, it all starts with talking to Him. Make your request and give thanks for what you do have. We all eventually need to find a relationship with a higher power. Whether it be today, next year, ten years from now, or near our death or the death of a loved one, we all eventually need that connection and support. The sooner you find that relationship, the better your odds of relieving your stress. By putting faith in a higher power, you can take the burden off your shoulders.

We don't always get what we ask. Sometimes one door closes, and another opens. In our case, if God had healed my daughter in the first year of her issues, I never would have learned this information that has enabled me to help other women struggling with similar issues. I was redirected from living a high-stress real estate broker lifestyle and worrying about closing the next sale to being a mother focused on helping her child. This led me down a path to share the inequities of today's treatment of women in modern medicine. God has His plans for each of us, but at the time it is happening, it's surely difficult to understand or see them.

Moving Forward

Letting go of past trauma does not mean condoning what someone did to you or your loved one. It does mean you no longer allow that person or event to occupy space in your mind or body. We accept that it cannot be undone but resolve to let it go. For events involving abuse or trauma, there's no question that qualified professional help can be beneficial and sometimes necessary. Do not be afraid to ask for help when it's needed. The only thing I caution here is to stick with your principles of no mind-altering drugs in place of natural treatments. There are holistic, natural-leaning psychiatrists and psychologists; while they aren't nearly as numerous as the standard psychiatrist, their numbers are growing.

A final thought on dealing with what is happening in our lives to create stress. There's no question it's important to spend time on yourself in dealing with relaxation techniques. However, it's also important to adopt an empowering mindset that makes a vow to find a way to accept and live with what is. Those with the most health issues are those who tend to have the poor-me mindset. We sow what we reap. If a person doesn't like where they are, there's the old adage that you have three choices:

1. Live with it.
2. Change it.
3. Change how you react to it.

We can say we have no choice in the current situation, and I surely agree in some instances. For example, when our daughter was in the emergency room multiple times per month during the same time period I was caring for my mother who had terminal cancer. I couldn't change the current situation. While we are stuck with the situation, we have two ways to deal with it. We can allow the effect on us to be health damaging by adopting poor stress-control habits, which is what it was for me when I chose to drink a glass or two of wine with snacks each evening to relax. Or we can do our best to support our body and mind during these difficult times. A better choice for me would have been some gentle exercise (no strenuous workouts to strain our adrenals during times of stress) with well-rounded meals. I made the choice; I paid the price. The health issues I dealt with in my late forties were a result of my actions in the years leading up to that time. The same principle applies to each of us. Take good care of the body you were given so that the body and mind are in better condition to deal with the stressors in your life.

It's also important to avoid negative thoughts. We go where our thoughts our focused. Each time we repeat a negative aspect of our life, our *brain* relives the experience, which means your *physical body* relives it. Just watch someone discuss something upsetting and observe their whole being get upset all over again. My mother's oft-repeated line was, "It is what it is." She raised ten children with an alcoholic husband. If anyone had the right to complain, it was her. And yet, I rarely heard her say a negative thought. She put one foot in front of the other on the bad days, as each of us has to do, and eventually the situation changed. When something upsets you, ask yourself, "Will this matter one year from now?" (or even one week from now).

The choice is accept, dwell on it, or change it. Some people look at bad health as bad luck. To accept it as bad luck is to accept remaining where we are. While I never imagined life could change regarding Karly's health issues to the degree it did, it came to the point we could not continue to sit back and accept the treatments she was given. Therefore, we had to investigate the *why* of her condition and make the appropriate change. Nobody could do it for us. Accepting what was and lamenting the situation wouldn't have changed what was happening. The choice was to consider what the current situation was and make the attempt to change it. We make our own luck. As my friend George would say, "You aren't lucky; you were blessed." I couldn't agree more!

Chapter Nineteen: Movement and Digestive System Care

Getting up and moving is one of the greatest things we can do for our mental health *and* our physical health. We want a nice physical workout that gets our heart rate up, builds muscle, and makes us breathe deeply. Remember, hard, intense, cardio workouts or marathon running is the opposite of what most young women (and older women) today should be doing. Most times this type of exercise will do more damage than good. Why? We have discussed them, but it's well worth repeating.

- Hard cardio causes the body to sense stress and signal the adrenals to supply us with elevated cortisol. We can go into a lengthy discussion of why chronic elevated cortisol is undesirable for us but, for our purposes, the main issue is the stress and demands cortisol production places on the adrenals. As an added incentive for avoiding intense workouts, note that belly fat cells contain four times more cortisol receptors compared with other cells. If you want to avoid the belly fat, avoid elevated cortisol.

- Stressed adrenals cause pregnenolone steal, which interferes with the production of pregnenolone and progesterone—both vital for normal female hormone balance.

- High cortisol levels are followed by high insulin levels, and invariably, we pack on the pounds.

A good alternative to intense cardio or marathons is something called peak training. You can view the information on Dr. Mercola's website at www.mercola.com. Peak fitness is a form of high-intensity exercise that

287

offers superb benefits to your overall health. It's a type of interval (anaerobic) training where you alternate short bursts of high-intensity exercise with gentle recovery periods. In comparisons to intensity training, the results were as good with less time involvement and less stress on the body.

It really comes down to doing something that gets your blood moving at least every other day—if not every day—of the week. Some people have better luck committing to a gym membership. Some prefer working out at home. Some do much better with a workout buddy, but you must be sure your workout buddy is motivated or all he/she will do is help give you reasons to skip today's exercise. I find it much easier to exercise at home. To me, it has great benefits *if* you are disciplined. I don't have to drive anywhere. I can exercise whenever it fits into my schedule, and I don't have to worry if I look like the ugly stepsister from Cinderella because nobody is going to see me. If I have to take time to look presentable every time I exercise, I would give it up. Therefore, the old "keep it simple" method has worked for me over the course of thirty-five years (off and on but mostly on). It's easier to be disciplined if you don't commit to difficult and lengthy exercise programs. But...you do commit to some form of exercise at the very least every other day. Hand weights are great for firming arms and getting the heart rate going. Throw the music on high with some fun tunes and warm up with dancing; dance like nobody's watching! (Hopefully, they aren't.) Then use the weights, some pushups (the girly kind are acceptable if your goal is maintain rather than "beefing up"), and end with some good stretching. It feels good; it gets the blood going and, most importantly, it's simple so it's easy to commit. Of course, on a gorgeous day, a good fast walk can replace the dancing. Get out and get fresh air as much as possible. Most of all, try to find something you enjoy whether it's dance, yoga, a structured exercise class, weights...whatever works for you.

The Benefits of Exercise

Circulation

You need and deserve time to help the body de-stress and receive good blood flow to help cleanse and regenerate. Circulation is an obvious answer and, unquestionably, vital to good health. If we are going to help the liver do its job of clearing bad estrogen, for instance, it needs to have blood flow. The same applies to all body systems and organs.

Lymph System

Another big benefit of exercise and movement is for our lymph system. Ladies, we can spend all the money in the world at the beauty counter, but if we don't get the lymph system moving, the bags under our eyes and our skin appearance is not going to be a pretty picture. Our circulation system has the heart to pump all our blood throughout the body and organs. But the lymph system has no heart and three times the fluid as the circulatory system. What pumps the lymph fluid? Our breathing and movement. Thus, the importance of taking deep breaths as well as exercising.

Detoxing

Finally, exercise makes us sweat. As we know, sweat isn't so good on your way to church but when you are exercising, it's awesome. Sweat is part of the body's overall detox system. If we don't detox, guess who is left picking up the ball? Your overworked liver. As we have discussed, your liver is on absolute overload on the toxin meter. If we don't move around and help it out, the excess estrogen hormones that were supposed to leave the body, remain in the body—not a good thing. Sweating is one way to detox. The other main ways are through excretion and deep breathing. What are some additional ways to help with body detox?

Detoxing the Body

Epsom Salt Baths

Far too many ladies forget when they are feeling awful from a bad menstrual period or a bad day that Epsom salt baths are great for detox. They add natural magnesium to the body, which is excellent for muscle relaxation. Hop in the tub and soak for at least fifteen minutes just prior to bed. If you are an essential oils user, add some lavender, majoram, frankincense, or whatever is your favorite to the Epsom salts prior to adding them to the bath. (This keeps the oils from floating on top the water in one puddle.)

Coconut Oil Pulling

This is an ancient practice that helps pull toxins from the body through the membranes in the gums and mouth. Swishing organic, unrefined (only use unrefined and organic) coconut oil for about fifteen minutes first thing in the morning is a great way to help the body rid itself of some toxins. This takes some pressure off the liver, and it's also great for gum health and whiter teeth. When you first start this habit, I find it's much better to start with less than the recommended amount of coconut oil (around one tablespoon). I would start with one teaspoon at first or else your jaws might get sore and you quit. You also don't need to go the full 15-20 minutes at first. Start out with 5-8 minutes so, again, the jaw doesn't get too tired. I find if I put this in the mouth right before I jump in the shower, the job is done. If I wait, it doesn't get done. After swishing, spit the coconut oil (full of toxins) into the wastebasket. Do NOT swallow it. After a quick rinse with fresh water, you are on your way. For detailed instructions, just Google coconut oil pulling and you will get a ton of hits with instructions.

Dry Brushing

Dry brushing involves a soft bristle brush that you brush in light strokes up each leg and arm then over the trunk of the body—all in the direction toward your heart. This is great for stimulating the lymph system, which ultimately helps with toxin excretion, and as a bonus, it's great for cellulite. This makes sense since cellulite stores toxins. When we stimulate the system to remove toxins, we don't need that nasty cellulite. Many of the bath and body stores as well as Amazon or other online retailers sell dry brushes that will come with instruction for dry brushing.

The more we detox, the more we take the burden off overworked organs so that they can do their job of achieving homeostasis (balance). A key in all of this is to eat right and stop adding in new toxins each day with junk food and chemically laden personal care and cleaning products.

Digestive System Care

We have already covered this topic extensively. Since we are discussing hormone health, however, I want to briefly review the importance of our gut health on our hormone health. Something we never learned in school (and neither do our doctors) is how intertwined our gut, hormone, and mental health are. Remember, as our gut health goes, our hormone health goes. If we have gut inflammation, we have whole body inflammation. That would include our overworked liver (again!), thyroid, adrenals, and ovaries to name a few. How can our glands secrete hormones at normal levels if they are inflamed? The digestive system encompasses the square feet of one full tennis court in our bodies, remember? If that amount of space is inflamed, you can bet the endocrine system is not functioning properly.

Along with the endocrine system issues, our moods are affected by this inflammation. I too often have mothers asking if I have suggestions for their children, parents, or teenage daughters. It seems more and more often, women in their twenties and thirties are struggling with anxiety, depression, and even panic attacks. As we talk about the gut health connection, sometimes a light bulb goes off in their head. They understand the connection. Other times, I get a vague look as though that can't possibly be the cause, and that makes me concerned. Not because I'm worried they don't trust what I'm saying (it happens occasionally!), but because this person will continue to struggle with trying a multitude of potentially risky options or treatments when it's unlikely she will get to the root cause until gut health is addressed.

How to care for our digestive system is covered in the first section. I hope you will read through it thoroughly. In this upcoming section we will discuss some shopping tips with the ultimate goal of learning a tad more on what's good and what's bad. We've had enough bad in our lives; let's aim for the good!

Chapter Twenty: Healthy Diet

"Apparently, you have to eat healthy more than once to get in shape. This is cruel and unfair."

This statement gave me a good chuckle. I'll admit I stole it from a meme my sister posted on Facebook. While it made me laugh, it's all too true that eating well must be a daily habit if we want to change our health for the better. Eating healthy really does get a bad rap for being bad tasting and unsatisfying, which is not true. It does eventually get where eating healthy tastes good and *feels* good. You will find if you eat junk for a day or two, you really want that salad or brown rice with grass-fed chicken instead of mashed potatoes and a commercially raised slab of meat. Really. Eating healthy is not about starving. It's about replacing bad with good.

When we eat food, we have vitamins, enzymes, amino acids, and lipids (to name a few) all working in synchronicity with each other to bring the body cell what it needs. One constituent may help deliver more efficiently to the cell receptor, and one may contain the nutrient the cell needs. Another may help retain cell fluid balance for better delivery. Thousands of processes and interactions are happening within the body as food is digested and constituents are delivered. Nothing can ever, ever, *ever* replace wholesome, healthy food. When we eat this healthy food, more of these various constituents are delivered to the body, and you will eventually feel more energy. Your hormones are able to synthesize properly, your brain is able to handle stress more effectively, and the inflammation in your joints is lessened. The list goes on. The next time you order mac & cheese or grab a donut, think about the consequences...because there *will* be consequences. And we have no one to blame but ourselves. We know what needs to be done.

Making the Change

Here's where working on self-speak comes into play. Start each day having a little chat with yourself. Encourage yourself, push yourself, and reinforce in your mind what you need to do for the benefit of yourself and your family. Change is not easy. That's a fact. People resist change. We like our daily habits. Decide whether those tiny little bodies you hug each day as well as your own body are worth making a change. You are the influencer, the teacher, and the parent of your children and yourself. Let' take a look at moving onward and upward on *how* to begin making that change (or continue if you already eat healthy).

We often see lengthy lists of what to eat and what not to eat. I will provide some suggestions of this later in this section, but for now, let's discuss getting started to healthier eating in your household.

Start at the Grocery Store

Look for *real* food, not food-like products. If it comes in a box or a bag, it *has* been processed. Any food that has been processed has preservatives (aka chemicals) to make it last longer and has had at least some if not many of the nutrients damaged or removed. Processing is just that—processing. When we process, we change, add, or remove. And in this day and age of manufacturers wanting to pump out cheap, attractive food, all holds are off as far as the chemicals they will use to provide it. Therefore, if you find food with a paragraph of ingredients, put it back. If you find a food that has a list of words you can't pronounce, put it back. If the first, second, or third ingredient is some form of sugar, put it back. It will be frustrating at first because you will be saying, "What the heck *can* I eat?" But getting tired of trying to figure things out is no excuse to give in and just buy what you are used to buying. We'll list some possibilities later in this section of safer foods. For now, get these basics down before we move on to that info.

Beware Swapping Bad for Worse

We often want to replace bad stuff with good, so we might pick up sugar-free, fat-free, or gluten-free products. Once again, manufacturers know this is what consumers will look for, so there will be big print splashed across the package advertising these. My suggestion is turn over the package and start reading the ingredients. Inevitably, what happens is one bad ingredient is exchanged for another to produce these seemingly better foods. If it says "gluten free," "sugar free," or "fat free," think chemical storm. I find this to be pretty much true. You know the routine by now... put it back.

Download a Phone App

Remember marketers are masters at appealing to your emotional triggers with words like "natural" and "organic" and attractive labeling, yet there are likely still chemicals or loads of sugar in the product. Think Dirty or EWG's Healthy Living are apps that detail a product's toxins rating. EWG has great lists of the Dirty Dozen (worst for pesticides) as well the Clean 15 (those that are better) plus many other lists that help you in grocery shopping. These apps really are great because you snap a shot of the UPC code and get a rating from 1 to 10 on ingredient concerns, nutrition, and degree of processing. You can use these apps for personal care products as well as food.

You can also print lists to help you make decisions. Print a list from any of these sites (or any others you discover) to take shopping with you. A few great sites with simple lists and ideas for what's healthy versus what's not healthy include www.EWG.org, www.healthychild.org, www.mercola.com, and www.draxe.com.

Watch for Marketing Ploys

When you see Vitamin "x" added (where "x" represents whatever vitamin the manufacturer chooses to add and advertise) on a package, beware. A glass of orange juice with eight or more vitamins added still likely contains as much sugar as a can of soda. Just because there are vitamins does not mean it's healthy. In addition, synthetic nutrients (nutrients added) never work in synergy in the body like the nutrients working together in whole food. Use your list or app to help guide you.

Watch for Sugars

There are at least sixty-one different names for sugar listed on food labels. Packaged foods, once again, are the big culprits for added sugars. Look at it this way. Sugar is cheap. Sugar is addictive. People *like* sugar. So what are manufacturers going to do? Add sugar. And why wouldn't they? However, manufacturers need to go with whatever sugar source is cheapest or tastes best in that particular food. Therefore, they have sixty-one different sources for their supply resulting in sixty-one names. This makes label-reading a tough job. Once again, use your phone app to scan the UPC code or refer to your list from www.EWG.org or Think Dirty for healthy foods.

Shop Outside Aisles

A good rule of thumb is to shop the outside aisles of the grocery store for the healthier foods. The produce aisle should become your favorite area but keep the rule of 80 percent greens, 20 percent fruits in your head as you shop. Fruit is loaded with antioxidants and great vitamins and enzymes, but fruit is also loaded with sugar. If we want to make a change in insulin levels, we need to limit sugar—no matter what form or food it is in.

Avoid Hunger Shopping

Do *not* shop for groceries when you are hungry. Remember we are much more prone to eating anything and everything when we're famished! Plus, you will tend to buy more of the junk since it looks so much more appealing. If you are to the "I'm starving" level, it's twice as important to stay out of the store. If you buy it, you will eat it. Avoid being undisciplined by resisting hunger shopping. Another little tip is to toss down a teaspoon (or tablespoon if you are a veteran) of unrefined coconut oil before heading out to shop. This helps blood sugar remain level. When our blood sugar drops, we start scooping up the ice cream and chowing down on the cookies.

Leave Little Ones at Home

It's not easy for young mothers to get out of the house without little ones when they head out to get groceries, but it's important to go alone. At least until you get used to what is good food and what is bad food. There will likely be a fair amount of label reading and decision-making. If you are distracted or trying to appease an impatient or fussy child, it will be much harder to learn and deal with the frustration of label reading. Once you get

297

used to your new normal foods, it will be easier to have children accompany you to the store. However, for the first few visits upon making the vow to eat healthier, see if you can't leave the little ones at home.

Avoid Rushed Grocery Shopping

The same principle as having little ones with you applies here. Label reading has become a hide-and-seek game with the food company's marketing team. Their job is to appeal to you with slick labels, and identifying the bad stuff becomes a guessing game. They want you to shop with desires while you need to shop with rational thought for good choices. This means taking your time, especially the first few times to the grocery store as you incorporate healthy choices into your diet.

Avoid Canned Goods

The linings of canned goods contain BPA, which is a known estrogen mimicker. Don't invite xenoestrogen to come home with you.

Avoid Commercial Milk and Meat

What? No milk and meat? What's a person to live on? Unless you are willing to spend the extra money to buy organic and grass-fed, it's vital for your health to steer clear of these. It may be a big change to go without them, but honestly, the dairy and meat in the grocery store today are poster children for how to mess up a body. Think back to our discussion on this topic regarding the slick little statement on these labels that reads, "No synthetic hormones added." The marketing teams for the manufacturer know consumers don't want hormones. So they throw us off by claiming their products have "no *synthetic* hormones." By law, they can't add synthetic hormones so it's not like their advertising means they care about you and yours; it's because they legally can't add them. However, as we discussed before, six naturally occurring hormones *can* be used on the animal. These include estrogen, progesterone, testosterone...you get the idea. If these go in the animal (which they do), where do you think these hormones end up? In the milk (including all milk products) and meat.

Beware *"Whole Grains" or "12 Grains"*

These labels are used to advertise food as supposedly healthy. What is wheat? A grain. What is in wheat? Gluten. Therefore, whole grain crackers or breads contain one of our big no-nos: gluten. You may be positive you have no gluten issues. If you have even one single health concern, be it allergies, asthma, endometriosis, fibromyalgia, thyroid imbalance, ear or sinus infection, or any other issue, avoid gluten for two weeks and see if it clears. It has happened and can happen. It's a pleasant surprise when it does, and you deserve a big pat on the back for making the discovery that gluten reactions are almost always in a manner we would least suspect.

I like Ezekiel bread, which contain ancient grains. Ancient grains are much more digestible and less irritating to the gut. There's no argument from me that they are not as soft as your more common breads, but then again, bread in ancient times wasn't soft either. Soft, gooey bread is a result of processing and manufacturing that takes away the natural enzymes for digestion. Thus, the gluten issue for so many today. I find the best way for me is to toast it. That way, you don't notice that it's not as soft as standard breads. Ezekiel bread comes in a variety of flavors such as flax, sesame, English muffins, raisin, and more. This brand rates great on the EWG web, and that's a good thing.

Getting decent food really shouldn't have to be so difficult. But it is. So rather than give in and eat junk, learn to play the game (with the help of your friendly websites and phone apps) and do the best you can. The more we, as consumers, use our money to buy healthy, chemical-free foods, the more manufacturers will change their methods to give it to us. The almighty dollar speaks. It's not going to happen through our government as we see by the eleven chemicals banned in the United States versus the 1,328 banned in the European Union. We cannot wait for nor rely on the government. It's up to each of us to spend wisely and make the food companies accommodate our demand.

Empty Your Kitchen Cabinets of Junk

There's a reason I listed start at the grocery store prior to starting at home. Who wants to look at an empty fridge and cabinets? Nobody. If we have nothing to put in our kitchen cabinets, we will be much less likely to get rid of the junk. If you bring home healthy food (and lots of it, especially at first) to fill the fridge and cabinets, you are much more likely to get rid of the junk.

Discuss Food with Your Children

If you don't educate them while they are little, they will eventually grow up, leave home, and fall into the food manufacturers' marketing ploys and go for eating what's fast and cheap. They are also going to be bombarded with television commercials showing beautifully colored, unhealthy foods. When you talk "why" you eat what you are eating and involve them in the preparation, they begin to have an appreciation for healthy foods. Healthy diet and lifestyle will be one of the biggest gifts you could ever give your body and your child.

Plan Ahead

Unless you have a great organic restaurant nearby, avoid eating out. Restaurants have no choice but to buy and cook their foods to appeal to the masses. The masses want cheap prices and large portions. The only way to provide this is via processed foods with cheap (toxic) ingredients. This is hopefully something you already avoid or is going to become a thing of the past for you. Take your lunch with you when traveling or eat your lunch at work.

Make meals and lunches ahead. If you are going to cook up some chicken breasts (please only organic and grass-fed), rather than cook enough for one meal, cook enough for three meals. Cut up the extra and put it in meal-sized or lunch-sized portions containers; it makes for an easy, healthy lunch rather than eating at the nearby fast food or coffee shop. If you are rushed in the mornings as you head for work (who isn't?), plan ahead. Cut up veggies or fruit and put them in containers or your lunch bag ahead of time. If we don't have food made up and ready to go, we get overly hungry and fall in the trap of grabbing what's near because we are too hungry to worry about eating right at that point.

Products to Avoid

While there are many products and foods to avoid that can be located through the websites or phone apps, I want to highlight a few that I feel may make the fastest and biggest impact in your hormone and gut health balance.

Soy

Like many of our foods, soy—in its natural state (fermented soy)—is good for us. For centuries, Asians have been enjoying the use of fermented soy products (natto, tempeh, soy sauce) with good health benefits. The problem with today's soy is up to 90 percent of it is processed or unfermented. In addition, up to 94 percent of soy in the United States is GMO. Unfermented soy has permeated a tremendous number of food products, especially processed foods on today's grocery shelves. It is listed on our food labels as hydrolyzed vegetable protein, lecithin, starch, and vegetable oil. If you see soy, soybean oil, or soy in any form other than fermented, avoid it. Unfermented or processed soy is a major source of xenoestrogens. Pregnant women should never use soy and absolutely do *not* use a soy-based infant formula.

Diet Sodas

If I had to choose between diet or regular soda, I would have to go with regular. Mind you, they are both one of the biggest cause of health concerns so I wouldn't really want either of them *but* the artificial sweeteners in diet sodas are a sure way to hormonal (and whole body) havoc, in my opinion. Artificial sweeteners are what? Artificial. They are created in a lab. You know what that means, right? Chemicals. They contain documented, harmful chemicals in the form of artificial sweeteners. Our government, once again, totally drops the ball in protecting the consumer on this one. Artificial sweeteners have been linked to migraines, gut issues, breast cancer, kidney disease, Parkinson's disease... the list goes on. If you are drinking diet soda and/or using low-cal products, one of the most important things you can do for your health is get them out of your household before your children also become hooked on them.

Soda

If someone offered you almost ten teaspoons of white sugar and you ingested that granulated sugar one teaspoon at a time, it might hit home the amount of sugar each can of soda contains. Just because that sugar is dissolved in a liquid, does not make it any less damaging. I have to think long and hard whether I will even put a teaspoon of honey in a cup of tea. I cannot begin to imagine ingesting ten teaspoons of sugar. And that's just in one soda. Some people drink multiple sodas per day. No wonder we have health issues in this country! For now, make sure you or your child is not one of the consumers. The health issues that may be resolved just by discontinuing this one habit could be great. Remember our discussion on all the things sugar does? It annihilates liver health (where estrogens are cleared), elevates insulin (causing whole body inflammation), and destroys microbiome balance in the gut (where up to 80 percent of immunity is). This is a partial list of ramifications. If we don't want to watch our child take medicines or get injections, avoid sugar with soda being a big culprit.

Dried Fruit

Dried fruit is a big culprit in sugar content. Dried fruits load up the sugar content in the diet and do not equate to a healthy alternative. The bad (sugar) in this case does not outweigh the small amount of antioxidants you might get.

Sports Drinks

They are loaded with high fructose corn syrup, artificial colors and flavors, and genetically modified organisms. A 32-ounce sport drink contains, on average, over fifty grams of sugar—the same amount as a can of soda. Any vitamins in these drinks are synthetic derivatives difficult for the body to recognize or break down. See my electrolyte recipe near the end of this chapter for a better option.

Health Drinks

Check www.ewg.org for any drink marketed as 'healthy'. Naked 100% Juice Smoothie Green rates at 6.2 with a 1 being great and a 10 being awful. Therefore, for something that should be healthy for us, a 6.2 is pretty dang poor. This juice contains thirteen teaspoons of natural sugar in one 15.2-ounce bottle. This is how it seems to go with almost all of the health drinks. While I'm sure there are a few that are decent, more often they are not. Use your trusty phone app to guide you through the maze of juices and drinks on the market. The best bet, of course, is a freshly made organic green drink made at home or a health store from fresh, organic vegetables with a small amount of fruit, if desired. Green juice does not store well as the natural enzymes in vegetables break down quickly. Thus, drink it shortly after making it and be aware most bottled health drinks add preservatives to avoid this fast breakdown of the nutrients.

Teflon or Nonstick Cookware

According to Dr. Mercola,

> Researchers found that the individuals with the highest PFOA concentrations were more than twice as likely to report current thyroid disease. PFOA and other chemicals are used to create heat-resistant and non-stick coatings on cookware. Studies have

linked these chemicals to a range of health problems, including thyroid disease, infertility in women, and developmental and reproductive problems in lab animals (**www.mercola.com**).

Search the Internet for articles and information to research the cookware that will best serve you and your family's needs as well as being safe.

Artificial Sweeteners

Avoid these especially if you are pregnant. Ladies, I cannot emphasize enough the dangers in artificial sweeteners. Pouring a chemical down your throat in the form of an artificial sweetener is a dangerous health assault to your body. No amount of supplements, oils, and even healthy foods can maintain health on a body being poisoned. Would you pour nail polish down your throat? No. Would you willingly ingest insecticide? No. Just because marketing and colorful packaging claims it's safe, there are a multitude of studies proving otherwise. 'Safe' does not make it safe.

We need to take off the blinders and research this subject before believing the FDA is protecting us in this matter. The approval process and the ties between the FDA and the manufacturers of these poisons is a revolving door of good ol' boys helping each other out at the expense of the average consumer's health. This includes and especially means diet sodas. It does not matter what the artificial sweetener is named. If it is an artificial sweetener, it is a chemical or foreign substance unrecognizable to the body—literally. Remember our discussion on this thought? If it's foreign to the body, it does damage to the body. The biggest culprits are:

Aspartame

According to Dr. Mercola, "85 percent of all complaints registered with the FDA are for adverse reactions to aspartame" (mercola.com). It is linked to migraines, seizures, kidney disease, brain tumors, and more. Aspartame is metabolized inside your body into both wood alcohol (a poison) and formaldehyde. "How aspartame was approved is a lesson in how chemical and pharmaceutical companies can manipulate government agencies such as the FDA" (www.mercola.com). It is found in NutraSweet, Equal, Spoonful, Equal Measure, and others in many popular diet foods and beverages. Aspartame was denied approval by the FDA three times.

Sucralose (in Splenda)

This is another dangerous artificial sweetener. Animal studies have linked it to increased male infertility, spontaneous abortion, and calcified kidneys.

GMOs (genetically modified organisms)

Shouldn't the name "genetically modified organism" be enough to tell us something is just not right about a GMO food? The top foods in the United States that are GMO are corn, soy, beets, and cotton. The seed of a GMO plant is created and *genetically modified* in a lab to be resistant to the chemicals used in weed killers growing around the plant. Weeds are some of the most resilient, intelligent greens on the planet. As they are sprayed with more and more chemical weed killer, they adapt to be resistant to it. Over time, more chemical spray equals more resistant weeds. The merry-go-round of "let's try to drown, burn, and destroy the resistant weed with chemicals" continues with the weed getting stronger each year. Thus, it requires more chemicals each year. The crop standing in the middle of these weeds being sprayed with increasing amounts of chemicals will end up in the food that goes on your dinner plate, your child's dinner plate, and likely your pet's food dish. The theory is the chemical will break down prior to being ingested. Our aforementioned gut health statistics and numerous studies say otherwise.

Glyphosate, the active ingredient used in these weed killers has permeated throughout farming systems not just in the United States but worldwide. Note this startling (and horrifying) information from a paper published on Feb 2, 2016 by Charles Benbrook, PhD, titled "Trends in glyphosate herbicide use in the United States and globally." He says, "Enough glyphosate was applied in 2014 to spray over three-quarters of a pound of glyphosate active ingredient on every harvested acre of cropland in the U.S., and remarkably, almost one-half pound per acre on all cropland worldwide." The same company that created this weed-resistant seed is the very same company selling the chemical to be sprayed on the crops. It's a built-in profit machine for the chemical company. But for you and your family? It's a gut-destroying, hormone-disrupting disaster. The familial coziness of the chemical company boards and our government legislators means we are not seeing legislation to prohibit this annihilation of our food system. Do you see how backwards this is? While the chemical companies rack up billions in sales, you and I and every single family who wants to avoid health-destroying chemicals have to pay *more* for organic food than conventional foods. Isn't it ironic that conventional is the label used on chemically sprayed foods? In the old days, organic would be conventional food and if something had chemicals sprayed on it, there would have been a big skull and crossbones across it. How greatly things have changed... and not for the better.

GMOs are banned or required to be labeled in over sixty countries. There's a reason they are prohibited, and anyone who ever tries to convince us that GMOs are safe is either totally misinformed or part of the GMO profit chain. Therefore, it's up to us to purchase organic if we want to avoid the chemicals. Avoiding GMOs or buying non-GMO foods is, once again, much more than a tree-hugging mentality. It is ultimately about survival and getting back to health, as our grandparents knew it before cancer became such a scary statistic.

We cannot continue to look at the price of organic food and eliminate it. To do so will continue the production of the chemically laden conventional foods. Yes, organic will cost more (which is a shame). Yes, organic produce will not look as full and pretty as the conventional stuff. But in most cases, you will notice a big improvement in flavor of the organic produce over the plumped-up, colorful vegetables and fruits. And honestly, change in our food system will not happen unless we make it happen by supporting the healthy stuff and refusing the cheap chemically infiltrated stuff. Whether it's bright colorful beads or apples, cheap cannot be our determining factor. In the meantime, get involved in writing or petitioning your legislators and vote for those (if you can find some) who support the small farmer and clean products.

Medical Tests

These need to be considered carefully. Medical tests done on females (and all people today) in our medical system are routine with little warning to the patient or consideration to the potential damage or chemicals involved. All tests involve at least some potential risk or chemical with hoses or needles being stuck in the body along with chemicals injected or through an IV drip.

Things like CAT scans and mammograms submit you to high levels of radiation. For our family, we asked, "What will you do if you find something?" before any tests. If the answer was to prescribe a med, we most often refused. If a medical test gives you a clue as to where to focus your research and support for your body, the benefit may outweigh the risks. But weigh carefully the cause and effect of medical tests. If you question at the clinic or testing center, you may or may not be well informed of the potential risks but more often than not, because tests are considered routine these days, you will likely be assured the risks are minimal. Again, do your research and also check natural health sites—not only medical sites—for discussion in the area of the test you are considering.

What to Eat

About now, I imagine you feel like saying "Superb. I can't eat, drink, or *do* anything." The number of things to avoid can be overwhelming, so let's get away from the no-nos and look at what we can and should do to help us have a healthy, well-functioning female body. Remember to review the list of health foods in the gut health section of this book and incorporate them with these suggestions. Many of those suggested in gut health are the same you see here for hormone health; this is emphasizing, once again, how most of the same foods and drinks support multiple body systems so we really only need to learn one good, overall, healthy diet plan.

Cruciferous Vegetables

This is equally important for young and older women alike. Every age is exposed to bad estrogen. Helping the body clear the bad, makes room in the receptors for our natural estrogen. Cruciferous veggies have a whole host of health benefits including sulfur and indole-3-carbinol, which bind to xenoestrogens to help the body break down and excrete them (alleluia!). This makes battling the xenoestrogens a little easier. Cruciferous veggies, such as broccoli, cauliflower, Brussels sprouts, kale, and cabbage also offer great support to our liver. That makes sense when we consider the liver is where our estrogens are broken down to be excreted. Studies increasingly indicate that dietary indole-3-carbinol (I3C) prevents the development of estrogen-enhanced cancers including breast, endometrial, and cervical cancers. Go for the cruciferous veggies. If that doesn't give you the relief you need, then consider supplements such as SAM-e that follows a similar function as cruciferous veggies. And remember, if you are going to load these veggies with Ranch or some other substance to help you get your veggies into your body, I'm afraid the bad will outweigh the good. Make up your mind to get used to the flavor of the veggie without any of the bad stuff on it. A squeeze of fresh lemon with some sea salt or Himalayan salt makes for a heck of a good snack once you get used to it.

Phytoestrogens (plant estrogens)

There are two sides of the coin on this topic with some saying plant estrogens contribute to high estrogen and thus, cancer. The problem I have with most of this research is it has been based on unfermented soy, which is processed soy. Considering 91 percent of soy and soy products in the United States are GMO, unfermented soy should be a big NO anyway. There is no question unfermented soy can contribute to multiple health issues and cancers. If we negate the studies on fermented soy, however, it takes out the majority of the studies showing negative effects of phytoestrogens on our health; rather, it shows studies that demonstrate their potential benefit. The theory on natural, plant-based phytoestrogens is these compounds bind to the same estrogen receptor sites on cells' xenoestrogens. They compete for the space on the cell receptor. When a receptor site is already occupied by a phytoestrogen, xenoestrogens cannot attach to it.

The great thing about phytoestrogens is they are tremendously weaker—gentler—in their estrogenic effects than xenoestrogens or even the body's more potent natural estrogens. So theoretically, phytoestrogens help protect the body against excessive estrogen stimulation by binding receptor sites against more potent xenoestrogens.

Phytoestrogens are found in all legumes, whole grains, flax seed, anise, black cohosh, and dark green leafy vegetables. I consume phytoestrogen-type plants with no ill effect, and I find they support my health. I feel good, and it appears these phytoestrogens are offering great estrogen balance support. Each person needs to look at the research and make your decision and, once again, be sure to look at research from natural health websites/articles for this information when making your decision.

Juice or Blend Fresh Veggies

Green drinks are excellent body cleansers. I often have people tell me I need to post recipes for my green drinks (or put some in this book). The problem is there is no recipe. I grab whatever I have in my fridge (and I make sure there is always a load of greens) and toss them in the blender or through the juicer. I personally don't worry about having any type of milk, such as almond or coconut milk, to add to it like some people. I use good old water as my liquefier. Now, I'm not going to brag about the taste of my green drinks, but here's how I look at it. It's going down the hatch regardless of the taste. I will agree it helps if it tastes good, especially for your children.

But sometimes what's in my fridge doesn't make the tastiest combination.

If it's green, eat it raw, blend it, or juice it but get some in your body daily. Be really honest with yourself (nobody else is going to know the answer). How many greens have you had today? Yesterday? Any day this week? Again, if you have some veggies cut up and ready to go in your refrigerator, your odds of ingesting, blending, or juicing some daily goes up greatly.

People want to start up the practice of blending or juicing but, by far, the bulk of the content in what they use is fruit. This does not count as a green drink. Walk the produce section, look for organic as much as possible, and load your cart. Get in the habit of loading up the juicer or blend at least every other day (to start). Throw in a little fruit if you must, but the majority should not be fruit.

What is the difference between juicing and blending?

- Juicing: You will get more veggie juice per serving by far but no fiber. I have heard of people using the fiber that comes out of the juicer in their muffin recipes, but I'm not quite that clever so you'd have to Google that topic. You could also compost the leftover fiber.

- Blender/blending: You get the fiber but less juice per ounce.

Both juicing and blending are great, and a combination of the two would be perfect. I currently have a blender with an organic store nearby that makes a great green juice. Therefore, I blend at home and swing by the organic store for juice occasionally. Many people find the juice more palatable to begin with, but a juicer usually costs more than a blender and might involve more clean up.

Healthy Cholesterol

Cholesterol is vital to proper hormone synthesizing. We have been ingrained by commercials and doctors to avoid cholesterol. This is a major health mistake that continues to perpetuate at the cost of American's health. When we block or interfere with cholesterol production, we interfere with normal body interactions. Cholesterol comes in the form of fish or animal fat, butter, ghee, fish oil, eggs, fish, and full fat dairy to name some of the top sources.

Our brain is the most cholesterol-rich organ in the body. When we have issues like depression, anxiety, dementia, we have to consider that cholesterol is a vital part of brain interactions. Today's women—both young and old—are greatly lacking in cholesterol either due to poor diet/processed foods or cholesterol meds. Think of cholesterol as the oil for your car. If the oil gets full of sludge (toxins and sugars), it's not the oil's fault. Therefore, when we ingest sugar, alcohol, bread, pastas, and sodas, it's not the cholesterol clogging the vessels—it's the sludge of toxins clogging up our vessels.

Therefore, throw the idea of avoiding cholesterol right out the window. (I'll throw in the caveat for my protection of "check with your doctor" on discontinuing any cholesterol meds or ingesting cholesterol rich foods/fats). What you do want to avoid is that bag of potato chips, crackers, cookies, or other packaged foods containing trans fats that cause inflammation in the vessels leading to cholesterol buildup in the veins. Inflammation in the vessels equals inflammation in the brain. High cholesterol in serum tests is more about inflammation in the body than it is about ingesting badly needed cholesterol. Blocking production of our natural cholesterol is an interference with a normal body process that is a recipe for disaster. For more on this topic, visit www.mercola.com and enter cholesterol in the search bar. This will bring up multiple articles—all extremely well researched and documented—on the risks of blocking cholesterol, why we need it, and the risks of health issues from using cholesterol medications.

Replace Table Salt with Himalayan or Sea Salt

There is nothing good in our table salt today, and that includes the salt placed on most restaurant tables. With America's awful habit of processing everything, table salt is refined and processed. Worst of all, part of the processing includes bleaching, adding chemicals to avoid clumping, and removing any beneficial minerals. I seriously wonder what goes on in the heads of the people who come up with these recipes for our foods and seasonings. When your doctors or health articles warn about avoiding salt, they are absolutely right when it comes to table salt. However, I would not avoid Himalayan and sea salt. Both are unrefined (think "unmessed with"), have excellent minerals, and they aid in creating beneficial enzymatic reactions in the digestive system. There are some slight differences between Himalayan and sea salt, but both are good and taste excellent.

Apple Cider Vinegar (ACV)

Add a small amount to water prior to meals to aid in digestion as well as occasionally throughout the day (about 1 teaspoon to 8 ounces of water) for a refreshing, pH-balancing drink. (I like the Bragg's Apple Cider Vinegar.) There are some great benefits from ACV:

- Helps maintain blood sugar levels (great for hormone support)

- Increases satiety
- Avoids hunger attack two hours later (due to blood sugar support)

Water

Fill three big bottles and set them on the kitchen counter each day. By the end of the day, make sure you have drank at least that much water. Nothing helps filter the kidneys, liver, tissues, and all body parts of chemicals better than water. In addition, it's the absolute best hydrator for the body on earth.

Healthy Fats

These should make up one-third to one-half of our daily calories. I know this seems a tad extreme, but more and more research shows the benefit of healthy fats (called saturated fats) as beneficial to inflammation, joint health, brain health, and so many other benefits. Yes, ask your doctor but remember you are now the specialist of your health; do not rely solely on this one person's advice. Do your research online (I always love www.mercola.com for well-researched and documented info) and natural health sites as much—or more—as medical sites. Examples of healthy fats are listed below.

The following is a very brief list for hormone support foods/compounds. It is far from a complete list because that would get overwhelming. Many of these are repeats from the gut health section, but they bear listing them separately in this area due to their importance on hormone balance. Therefore, I will touch upon the highlights of what I use and suggest. All products suggested are organic (not standard, commercial foods). This will hopefully give you some ideas of foods to look for. From this point, research

315

and decide what is best for you and your family.

Cheat Sheet for Hormone Balance

THIS

- Good fats (coconut oil, hemp oil, fish oil)

- Butter, ghee, egg yolk, flax (phytoestrogen)

- Organic, grass-fed meats

- Organic, air-popped popcorn with butter and/or coconut oil and sea salt

- Eggs from organic, grass-fed, pasture-raised hens; cage-free, vegetarian, free-range (all better than commercial eggs but not as good as pasture-raised

- Basmati, Black or Brown rice, Quinoa

- Cruciferous Veggies (cauliflower, broccoli, cabbage, Brussels sprouts, kale)

- Himalayan or Sea Salt

- Apple cider vinegar or fresh lemon in water

- Stevia, Honey, Molasses, Maple Syrup

NOT THAT

- Canola, Corn, or Soybean

- Fat processed in oil

- Avoid GMOs and limit dried fruits

- Commercial meats labeled "no growth or synthetic hormones"

- Microwave popcorn (BIG no-no)

- 12 Grains, whole wheat, white, or any processed bread

- Agave (the high fructose content is worse than any commercial sweeteners)

- Packaged, gluten-free, sugar-free, fat-free products

- White Rice, Potatoes, Bread

- Table Salt

- Soda, Diet Soda, Sports Drinks, Juice Boxes, Bottled Juice

- Unfermented soy, soybean oil in processed foods like mayo, salad dressings, crackers, chips

316

My Food Routine

Below are a few ideas for foods that I eat that are considered healthy and have found helpful for hormone support. I realize what I eat may not fill up a hungry husband or some females used to more starches but they are a few ideas for adding to your eating plan. These are only a few suggestions. While they may not seem filling, I suggest grabbing and eating one of these when you're hungry. Then, if still hungry, at least you won't eat as much of the less healthy stuff.

Morning Coffee ("Bulletproof Coffee")

Are you a "straight up" black coffee kind of person? When I first tried bulletproof coffee, I was surprised I liked it even though it has some added (healthy) flavor. Why did I try it in the first place? Because it has some very excellent things in it for our body support, and I wanted to make my morning coffee more beneficial without ruining the taste of my favorite drink of the day. Here's the simple recipe:

- 1 Tbsp grass-fed butter (supporting our healthy cholesterol)
- 1 Tbsp MCT (medium chain triglycerides) oil or organic, unrefined coconut oil
- 1 drop liquid Stevia
- 1 cup of organic, dark roast coffee
- A pinch of baking soda to help neutralize the acid in the coffee

Mix all of the above in a large glass container. (I just use a large coffee mug and only fill about two-thirds full then finish filling with coffee once blended.) Use a hand-blender to mix/froth. This comes out looking and tasting like a cappuccino without the unhealthy ingredients. MCT oil is a derivative of coconut oil; but the process for MCT oil involves extracting and using the powerful portion of the coconut oil. You can get it from www.bulletproofexec.com, Amazon, or www.Thrive Market.com.

Breakfast

My favorite breakfast is comprised of:

- Cucumber slices with fresh lemon squeezed over them and Himalayan salt

- One egg (organic and from pasture-raised hens)

- Kefir breakfast blend

- Chia seeds, buckwheat groat, hemp seeds (all can be purchased individually and organic from Amazon or Thrive Market)

- Pour Unflavored Kefir (preferred instead of yogurt because yogurt has lactose) over three tablespoons of the above combo

- Add one scoop high-quality vanilla protein mix

- Add fresh or frozen mixed berries

- Add organic walnuts or pecans

- Add a teaspoon of powdered cinnamon

- Stir together and let seeds mixture absorb the liquid in the kefir for about five minutes.

I know the seed combo seems a tad back to nature, but I'm here to say it's kind of like your own homemade granola without all the cane syrup and oatmeal. I buy the three different bags of seeds/groat, pour them all together into one container and mix them together. From then on, all you have to do each morning is scoop out the three tablespoons into a bowl and add the rest. The seeds give great fiber and nutrients, the kefir is a great fermented food, and since it's a tad more watery than yogurt, I can add the powdered protein mix without it getting too thick. It really is much like yogurt and granola only much healthier and, once you get the bags of seeds/groat ordered and sent to you, it's super easy.

On alternate days, I go for a green drink and two eggs cooked up over easy and one slice of toasted Ezekiel flax seed bread.

Snacks

- Apple slices make a great snack. If it's organic, wash well and leave the skin. If not organic (apples are #2 on the dirty dozen), peel off the skin.

- Raw pumpkin seeds or sunflower seeds are great! I sprinkle some salt over them; sometimes it sticks, sometimes not, but it gives them a tad more flavor.

- A handful of Food for Life brand, Ezekiel Cinnamon Raisin cereal (rated a 2.4 on the EWG site/app)

- A scoop of Hemp protein mixed with water (Essential oils users, add a drop of cinnamon vitality oil and black pepper oil for flavor and absorption.)

- Fresh veggies with fresh lemon squeezed over it. Sprinkle with Himalayan or sea salt. Some of my favorites:
  - Cauliflower
  - Cucumber
  - Avocado
  - Red or green cabbage
  - Carrots (limit carrots due to high sugar content)

- Organic dried wolfberries are super great for antioxidants but don't get too carried away; like all dried fruit, the sugar content adds up.

- Cut up cheese: I like pepper cheese for a little bite plus the pepper portion of it helps with nutrient absorption of any accompanying food I have with the cheese. Have no more than about eight bite-sized pieces; cheese has lots of starch and yeast.

- A tablespoon of organic, unrefined coconut oil (off the spoon and into the mouth). This is great for curbing appetite (for those who crave sweets or watching calories, this is a great way to help), inflammation, and metabolism. Do *not* worry about calories on any of your healthy fats. They make up for any calories by supporting healthy metabolism.

- Soft-boiled eggs (overcooked eggs damages the nutrients and enzymes). The more raw, the better.

Lunch or Dinner

- Salad: A handful of organic mixed greens that comes in the plastic (ugh) tub at the grocery store with fresh lemon squeezed over it and Himalayan or sea salt sprinkled over top. Chop up the lettuce, throw in any other raw veggies that sound good, add some green olives, red onion, pumpkin seeds, and sunflower seeds. I also chop up some fresh Romaine lettuce and add it along with cut up organic, grass-fed chicken.

- Organic, grass-fed chicken: Cut up and mixed with basmati rice (or brown rice). Cooks like regular raw rice, no instant! Toss in raw carrot, celery, and garlic cloves near end of rice cooking time. Add organic chicken broth to keep it from getting too dry.

- Food for Life, Ezekiel 4:9, Whole Grain Pocket Bread (rated 1.7 on EWG site/app) with some sliced pickles, red onion, cucumber, organic, grass-fed sliced roast beef or turkey and cheese with chopped Romaine, Himalayan salt, and fresh ground pepper.

- Wild-caught salmon with fresh lemon, dinner salad, and cooked broccoli or fresh cabbage wedge with fresh lemon squeezed over them.

- Obviously a person couldn't exist on just these foods/meals and perhaps they won't feed a family, but hopefully a couple of them will work their way into other meals you make. I'm apparently not a great cook, so I eat loads of fresh stuff. If you are one who tends to cook, sautéed kale in coconut oil with garlic and lemon is a great healthy meal. Cauliflower crust pizza with healthy toppings is another good one as well as many more recipes available online. The point here was to give you a few ideas for getting started or adding to your existing meal plans.

Green Drink Ideas (ideally organic and well rinsed)

As I mentioned earlier, I put very little fruit in my green drinks. Too much fruit (even though good for us) is too much sugar. Fruits are easy to add to our diet through adding berries to oatmeal or kefir/yogurt, munching on an apple, orange, or banana. Veggies are a tad tougher for people to include in daily diet so throwing ample veggies in a green drink helps add them to the diet.

- Any type of greens: kale, cilantro, romaine, dandelion greens, sunflower or broccoli sprouts, parsley
- Whole turmeric root
- Whole Ginger root
- Hemp protein (protein fibers help bind to metals and carry them from the body)
- Hemp oil

- Beets or beet powder
- Carrots (limit due to sugar content)
- Celery
- Cucumber
- Whole lemon (one half lemon per green drink)
- MCT oil
- Pick one fruit (not all)-One half of an apple, orange, or banana, blueberries, strawberries or raspberries

Throw all in the blender and blend away to a tolerable consistency. It seems no matter how much I blend, mine stays fairly thick so you may want to add more liquid rather than blending the daylights out of it, which might ultimately affect the enzymes in your vegetables.

As aforementioned, green drinks do not store well. You can get away with refrigerating and using for around twenty-four hours but after that, the enzymes break down and start creating non-healthy constituents in the drink. I add plain water as my liquid, but some people like almond, coconut, or organic, grass-fed cow's milk. Just make sure your almond or coconut milk does not contain *carrageenan*—a natural thickening agent known to cause gastric distress and that your milk comes from organic, grass-fed cows.

Of course, you can add anything you want to your drink. Experiment and see what you like and also what's available at your store or farmers' market. The key is to get some greens in your body. Keep it simple so you don't give up. Try to get a decent enough flavor that you will drink it. If you just can't get used to the flavor of green drinks, be sure you are cutting up some cucumbers, celery, and salad greens and eating them fresh. The biggest flaw in the American diet today is lack of whole greens.

Electrolyte Recipe

4 cups hot (not boiling) water

1/4 cup fresh lemon juice (not bottled Lemon juice)

1 Tbsp Bragg's Apple Cider Vinegar (ACV)

1 tsp raw honey

1/4 tsp sea salt or Himalayan salt

Dissolve honey and salt in hot water. Let cool slightly and add the ACV and lemon. Throw in your fridge and drink as needed. Personally I believe in drinking fluids at room temperature for best absorption so just pull it out shortly before your workout or before you need it and let it warm up slightly. This is not necessarily only to be used for people who exercise. The ingredients in this recipe make for a great refreshing drink any time of day.

Sum It Up

Something I find interesting about all of these lists. Our grandparents (great-grandparents for you younger ladies) did almost all of the things on these lists naturally without anyone discussing it with them. It was their lifestyle. And, if you look back at that time period, these women had lives that depended on their ability to do very physical work, which required a strong healthy body. They did not have time for cramping and excessive bleeding. They ate eggs and grass-fed meat; they had minimal chemicals in their environment. They had perhaps one sweet treat per day, and they surely didn't have birth control pills or synthetic hormones to manage their hormone health. They grew their own food so they didn't worry about chemicals such as glyphosate on their carrots or cauliflower. Thus, their generation lived with basic lifestyle habits greatly different in our world today. And they did *not* struggle in anywhere near the numbers we do.

Our world today is vastly different. Even worse, we have been convinced what a better world we live in compared to our grandparents. With modern conveniences, I'd say it is better. But when it comes to caring for the human body, we are failing miserably in comparison. We eat processed foods. We ingest or inhale chemicals and apply them to our body. We use synthetic hormones for birth control. We are warned (incorrectly) not to have cholesterol in our diets. We live stressful lifestyles, and our days are so crazy that fitting in even casual exercise is rare.

Our world today is a world of landmines to females—the female cycle, the female body, and the female person—we were created to be. We unknowingly were sucked into this vortex of sugar-laden diets then pills, chemicals then pills, and stress then pills. We learned it from our parents and from a medical system infiltrated by public enemy #1—the pharmaceutical world that has all of us brainwashed that the miracles of science are smarter than the miracle of creation and the awe-inspiring interactions within the human body.

It's not you. It's your hormones. But like it or not, you are stuck with them. They are powerful, and they are highly interconnected. If one is off, the chain reaction throughout the entire body is set off. Hormones are what make you a female. And, like it or not, we better figure out what makes them unhappy because when your hormones ain't happy... the entire body ain't happy.

So make changes! Don't worry about doing them all at once. Pick one positive thing you can do and do it. Take the time to search and search and search again until you find a health practitioner who really listens and agrees with a no-pill lifestyle and medical care. Join Facebook groups or other groups that have a like mindset as yours. Look for and interact with friends who have the same ideals so you can support each other. Groups are also a great resource for helping find products, stores, and health practitioners who lean toward natural.

When it gets bad enough, change will happen. Don't wait for it to be bad enough. Make changes before it gets to that point. Make change happen for you and make it happen for your family.

If not you then who? Who is going to clear out the chemicals? Who is going to introduce fragrance-free, clean products? Who is going to take the time to learn healthy versus non-healthy foods? Who is going to look around your home and make it your chemical-free safe haven? Just as important in all of this is the question... *who* is going to research and go toe-to-toe, if necessary, with a pharmaceutically ingrained doctor to insist on medical treatment that does not center around powerful prescription medications? In her book *Lean Forward Into Your Life*, author Mary Anne Radmacher states it well: "Courage does not always roar.... It is the quiet voice at the end of the day saying, 'I will try again tomorrow.'" Her preceding words make an excellent point on which we can build by knowing courage is taking care of you and yours. Tomorrow can start with saying no more. No more chemicals, no more influence of synthetic pharmaceuticals or over-the-counter prescriptions, no more junk food and high amounts of sugary treats. No more.

It's easy to say but a tad more difficult to implement. This is where your courage to take a stance comes in. Courage to remain with your newfound convictions and implement them even if you don't get the support at home, at work, or at the doctor's office. Set the standard and be the example for your family. Your courage will benefit not only you but the people around you as your healthy habits are implemented and observed. The influence of healthy habits goes well beyond any material gift you could ever give yourself or your loved ones. The changes you make will very likely make a great difference in your and your children's hormone balance as well as whole body health. This makes being strong and keeping your determination for change well worth it.

It takes effort, it takes energy, it takes conviction, and it takes courage. But isn't that what females have always done when the chips are down? Have no doubt, in today's world of environmental factors on hormone disruption and lack of medical knowledge for how to treat today's female, the chips *are* down. And you're the only one who can beat the odds for you and your family.

I believe you are up to the task... Now go out and roar!

Summary

"You're on your way and you know what you know. And YOU are the one who'll decide where to go." —Dr. Seuss

You're on your way! You have learned about the power of the gut on whole body as well as brain health. You have been given valuable information on the need to remove sugars and grains for your gut health *and* hormone balance. You've read about stress and its ability to greatly interfere with our hormone interactions. You are aware of the frightening damage from chemicals' insidious permeation into your environment through your personal care and cleaning products as well as your food.

A tremendous amount of information was presented with many suggestions for improving health for you and your family. Information is great. Now how do we use this information? I was recently asked a great question along this line. A lovely young lady asked me, "If you had to choose the one most important thing to change or use for health improvement, what would it be?" I know she wanted me to name a supplement or food or daily habit—the Holy Grail, so to speak—in answer to the question of health support that might make the biggest impact on her health issues. Honestly, it took me some time to respond to the question as I pondered all the possibilities.

Ultimately, if I had to choose the one most important thing I believe is necessary to use for health improvement in your life my answer would be to: *be aware*. Although this response may not be what she was looking for, I believe it's a fair answer. It is the one thing to incorporate into our lives if we are going to make a change for the better. Be aware of your habits, routines, what you use, eat, or do in life as you go through each day on autopilot. Slow down to be present in the moment as much as possible so you recognize what you are doing *as* you are doing it. What are your habits? There's no better time to become aware of an area to improve than when you are in that moment. Ask yourself what would be a better alternative?

Many of us are too comfortable in the environment we live. So if we do not become aware of our habits and environment, we go through each day with our same routines, same products, same foods from the grocery store, and same personal care products. How can we change our habits if we are not aware of them?

This possibly seems like a vague answer to a great question, but let me expand. Going through your entire kitchen, reading labels, and trying to determine good from bad can seem overwhelming—a job we will get to one of these days. However, if you pay closer attention (are more aware), you might notice as you scoop out macaroni and cheese onto our child's plate that this may not a good food choice. You are aware of what you are eating and feeding your child (good job!). As that thought occurs, stop and think what would be better. Quinoa or maybe brown rice with organic chicken broth as a base? Grab your grocery list and add brown rice and/or quinoa as well as chicken broth to it. It may be you don't know how to make quinoa or brown rice or if you even like it, but add it to the list. Buy it, get on the Internet, and choose easy recipes. Make it next time instead of macaroni and cheese. Bingo. You just made one good change because you were aware of the bad.

Be aware from morning to evening. As you start the day and jump in the shower to shampoo your hair, be aware of the strong fragrance that, in the past, you believe smelled great. Now you notice the smell, turn the bottle over, and see the word "fragrance" as the third ingredient with Sodium Lauryl Sulfate (SLS) as #1. Your shampoo has more chemicals than safe ingredients. When you get out of the shower, you grab your phone and add "safe shampoo" to your shopping list. You may not know a safe one or where to get it, but that's your next health mission. Following this plan of being more aware, you've already done two things within maybe a week (replacing macaroni and cheese and finding a safer shampoo).

Being aware means you notice the steaming hot water going through the thin plastic coffee pod, the lengthy list of chemicals in your sunscreen, the standard milk product in your fridge. Each time you notice, you add a healthy alternative choice to your list. Does this mean we have to become paranoid? No. And we can't use that as an excuse. It means making your choices where you want to change. But you can't make choices if you aren't aware and take notice of the bad in the first place. When you aren't aware, you continue to choose the old behavior, and you choose the consequences. If the behavior is unhealthy choices, that consequence may not be for only yourself. It will be for your children as well. Children are a sponge. They watch, they see, they learn. Monkey see, monkey do. Be aware.

Most of all, be aware daily habits *do* make a difference. Habits and routines count and add up to either health or illness, depending on whether you become aware of these habits and routines to acknowledge change needs to be made.

We are a lost generation. We lost our birthright of good health and clean environment by having chemicals in our food and environment introduced to us at birth. We learned to incorporate them into our daily routines, which gave us the impression they were safe and acceptable. We never suspected they were toxic to our bodies, mind, and soul. As we become aware, we make the decision to stand up to make a change. Because if we don't, we will have another lost generation: our children and grandchildren.

Be aware. Be cognizant. Be present in the moment so you can recognize where to incorporate change. Because, when you know better... you do better. Healthy choices make a healthy body. One step and one product at a time. You know what you know. Now *you* decide which direction you'll go.

If You Are Struggling...

There were many times I prayed for our daughter Karly's health. I would question God by asking, "Why does a good Christian girl have to suffer like this? Why does she have to be in such pain when she's so young and done nothing to deserve this?" Her continued decline in health coupled with her being a victim of a brutal physical attack and two devastating car accidents eventually made me question my faith. However, there came a time—a breaking point—when things were so bad I had to accept and turn everything over to God.

During my most difficult moments in trying to understand Karly's health issues, I heard a beautiful sermon that gave the advice for those struggling to "place our worries at the feet of God... and walk away." Continually making the same requests to Him demonstrates a lack of faith in His plans for us. This was my turning point. God knew what we so desperately wanted. But it wasn't His plan at that time. When the door does not open, it may not be, "No." It may be, "Not yet, you have some growing yet to do." Looking back, I now understand how significant this is. Being broken and humbled to learn we are not in control is a heartbreaking process. But it is necessary to bring us to the point of opening the door to a deeper relationship with Him.

I am humbled by God's wisdom and love. I am thankful for his direction to acquire healing for our precious child who, once so far gone, is now healed. Looking back, I see our struggles were a force in our learning. Learning that opened our eyes to how very wrong what we were doing was for the healing process we desired. Watching a child in pain provided the driving purpose that pushed me to look for and devour information for healing in the way He intended and designed.

I am forever grateful He led us in using the gifts of His wisdom and of the energy of this earth to help us find healing power in His way rather than continuing to turn our health over to a system that goes against His plan of the body and universe co-existing in benefit to each other. I feel blessed for the opportunity to reach out to others who are struggling in hopes of bringing His form of healing that works with our body rather than against His plan by interfering with our body.

We must ask God, that's true. But at some point, we must give things over with trust in Him and his plans for us. There is a passage from Philippians 4:6 that reads, "Be anxious for nothing, but in everything by prayer and supplication with thanksgiving make your requests be made known to God." Handing things over at the most difficult time in our life isn't easy, but it's what gets us through it. When we turn it over to Him and he shares our burdens, we no longer shoulder them alone. Instead, we find the comfort and strength we so badly need to help us through these times.

Part Three: Essential Oils

Disclaimer

The content in this book is for educational and informational purposes only, and it is not intended as medical advice. I am not a medical professional and cannot diagnose, treat, or prescribe. The information contained herein should not be used to diagnose, treat, prescribe or prevent any disease or health illness. The author and printer accept no responsibility for such use. Please consult with a qualified, licensed health care professional before acting on any information presented here. Any statements or claims about the possible health benefits conferred by any foods, supplements, essential oils, or lifestyle changes have not been evaluated by medical professionals or the Food & Drug Administration.

Chapter Twenty-One: The Essentials of Essential Oils

How do I love essential oils? Let me count the ways.... Using a pure and natural substance is the safest, least invasive way to work with our body. The aroma of a pure essential oil has the ability to soothe, unwind, relax. Essential oils contain plant constituents that are one of the greatest gifts God gave us to support this vessel within which we reside—the miraculous creation known as the human body.

This body of ours intuitively knows what feels good and what feels right in support of its natural ability to come to balance/homeostasis. When a constituent is natural and unadulterated, the cell receptors of the body can more readily recognize, absorb, and utilize what is offered. With essential oils, we like to say we offer to the body rather than force it to do what we (or something created in a lab) want it to do. The body knows how to come to balance—our job is to give it the tools to do so. Removing toxins and chemical disruptors, providing appropriate nutrition, and supporting with plant constituents in the form of essential oils is an excellent recipe for body systems balance.

Throughout this book, we have discussed the importance of eliminating hormone-disrupting and damaging toxins from our daily lifestyle and environment. There are many ways to use essential oils (EOs) to help eliminate chemicals and toxins. Personal care and cleaning products with essential oils provide a fabulous way to get started on the elimination process. Here are a few quick examples:

- Organic, unrefined coconut oil with some lavender or geranium (or both) EOs makes a wonderful body lotion. There are a variety of great recipes for body butters and lotions using natural products and a variety of essential oils. Choose which scent you attract to and use it. This means you no longer will be applying fragrance-ridden commercial lotions with a long list of chemicals in the bottle.

- Diffusing lemongrass smells amazing, and it is absolutely toxin/chemical free. There are hundreds of great combinations of EOs you can use to diffuse in your home or office. This makes a great replacement for the chemically laden plug-ins, candles, and sprays. Your entire home can still be filled with your favorite scent. This can also serve other purposes in addition to smelling great: to soothe, invigorate, inspire, and motivate. The choice is yours, and the array of choices is endless.

- My sun care lotion contains only coconut oil with lavender essential oil. I sometimes add carrot seed oil to the mix but often just the lavender oil. Not only is it all I use in the Florida sun with no ill effects, I'm also supporting great skin health when the sun warms my skin to open my pores and absorb the lotion. No chemicals to absorb into my pores and it supports skin health...a win-win!

These are only a few examples of ways to use essential oils in our lives to help eliminate chemicals and toxins. There are entire books of recipes as well as Pinterest and Facebook pages loaded with them. For the sake of space, I won't list recipes, but please know you *can* replace chemicals with natural products; there is an abundant supply of recipes available.

Replacing chemicals is so much more than a "maybe I should remove them" type of thing. The danger of chemicals not only to hormone disruption but also in contributing to cancer is huge. Something as simple as homemade products may seem as though it would not be helpful or important but the first time you or someone you love hears the words "cancer," you will do everything in your power to beat it, right? So let's do everything in our power right now. Removing chemicals is powerful. Finding chemical-free personal products is outrageously difficult. Making your own is outrageously simple and effective.

Imagine if you bring your little ones up from a young age to discuss the importance of avoiding chemicals and how you do this with natural products. They will be instilled with the importance of clean and pure rather than chemically laden products. This is truly one of the greatest gifts you could give them—the knowledge of respecting and caring for their body. It's a gift that will keep on giving for the rest of their life!

Now that we know EOs can help replace chemicals in our everyday products, what other ways can we use them? We can apply them topically, inhale, diffuse, and (for certain oils only) use internally for body systems support. What else can they do? If you are an oils user, you may already know most or all of the ways and whys. If you do not use essential oils, I recommend you absorb some of the information we will discuss as well as conduct further research into this area. If a person involved with EOs referred you to this book, please contact them to assist you in pursuing the many ways EOs can benefit your life.

EOs have impacted many lives in a positive, powerful way including mine and my daughter's health. Our results with a couple of EOs given to us by a friend (thank you, Diane Siemers!) first opened our eyes to the possibility of working with the body to offer it support. When we were at a very low point in our lives, she offered us lavender and lemon oils to uplift our mood. When I first sent these two EOs to my daughter at college, she texted me to tell me, "These oils stink. They don't smell good like the pharmacy oils." At that time, I didn't know much, but I knew pharmacy oils likely had synthetic fragrance (a chemical). I responded, "That's because the pharmacy oil has fragrance added, but that's not good so please use the EOs I sent you." So she did. After diffusing these oils for a few days, she texted me the following message: "These oils you gave me are amazing!" I was very pleasantly surprised at her comment. To be honest, I had gotten the oils to be nice to my friend who kept recommending them to us. I didn't actually expect any type of positive response, especially an emphatic response from someone who was already convinced she didn't like them. So, both she and I were surprised by their effect.

I'd like to say things were all good from that point on, but they weren't. We had a long way to go including the winding road of getting Karly to change her eating habits and toxin exposure. However, the EOs *did* open our eyes to their power for eliciting a positive response. And that's where my EO journey began. I devoured every bit of information I could to see what I could use to support our mental and physical health.

While both Karly and I had to work to recover our health through diet stress relief and chemical removal, we made these necessary changes with the result being we improved our health to the point we were now above the wellness line. Now that our health is above the wellness line, we love the support they give our body systems and particularly the systems involved in our focus in this book: the nervous, digestive, and endocrine (hormone secreting) systems.

Quality Over Cost

The use of essential oils has become a new fad lately with the sales exploding for nearly every oil company. They are sold everywhere from online to big box stores and pricing from what some people consider high all the way to extremely low at the large retailers or online. These oil companies include everything from well-established companies with decades-long reputations of safety and purity (Young Living) versus newer companies—some of which are jumping on the bandwagon—to cash in on the years of research and work done by the pioneers in this field. Thus, it's important for each person to study, research, and look for quality instead of letting price guide you.

Reputation and experience are important in the quality of an essential oil. Studies such as the 2015 abstract "In-vitro anti-cholinesterase activity of essential oil from four tropical medicinal plants" have "shown or demonstrated the considerable variability in the composition of the essential oil from different parts of the same plant." Thus, an oil may come from a more available part of the plant—say the leaf—when perhaps the root is, by far, the more potent and constituent-rich part of the plant. Taking it from the more available but less potent part of the plant means a company can produce more oil to deliver to the store or online. Since it's more available, the price can be cheaper. The more potent and effective part of the plant may not be as available thus will likely cost more. Potency and effectiveness are where the true value in supporting the body comes into effect. Therefore, cheaper is very likely not a good deal and, literally, can be dangerous should you choose to follow the common advice found online and elsewhere to use EOs from topical, inhalation, and diffusing to internal. If we are going to inhale, ingest, or apply a constituent topically, it's vital it be pure and safe.

The essential oils I refer to in my use of EOs are *only* Young Living essential oils. This is not to make a pitch for Young Living oils, but I am familiar with their use as well as their safety. I have used them for seven years and experienced their fabulous support. In addition, they own the farms from which many of their oils are harvested and distilled. What better way to control time of harvest than by owning the farms? I will list some things to look for when choosing your essential oil company as well as why I use Young Living essential oils. I cannot vouch for the quality of other companies, but I can vouch for Young Living since I have used them topically, inhaling, diffusing, and internally for seven years with no negative reactions and many positive reactions. Are there other good, high-quality companies? Yes, there are. However, I am not as comfortable and familiar with them as Young Living. So please, do not use the list below and go online or to your local store to purchase. My recommendation is not familiar with their quality or possible lack of quality. My experience and recommendations are only with using Young Living EOs. Throughout this section, when I refer to EOs I am referring to Young Living essential oils.

Now let's discuss why we need to respect the power of EOs. Oils are powerful! Did you know...

- It takes 256 pounds of peppermint leaf to make one pound of peppermint essential oil.
- It takes 75 lemons to make one 15-ml bottle of lemon oil.
- It takes 22 pounds of rose petals to make a 5-ml bottle of rose oil.
- One 15-ml bottle of lavender takes 27 square feet of lavender plants.

We must respect their power to support and their ability to do harm when used incorrectly.

In my writing on oils that support specific body systems as well as the EOs I personally use, you will occasionally see the words "vitality oil." Young Living has many oils approved for internal use. These oils are labeled as Vitality™ oils. When you see the word vitality on a bottle of Young Living, you will know it has been approved for internal use.

There is much discussion on the subject of EOs and internal use. My family and I have and do use them internally. We also respect the delicate balance of gut microbiome health as we have discussed at the beginning of this book. Some oils may support this balance while too much of most any oil can disrupt it. For this reason, I use EOs internally if I have a specific reason to do so such as occasionally using Peppermint Vitality Oil™ in a small amount of water after eating to soothe and support digestion. I use the minimum I feel is needed to support the system. I'm not a fan of recipes containing high amounts of EOs for internal use. Oils are powerful, and gut health is a fine balance of microbiomes and bacteria. My advice would be to avoid overuse internally and only when necessary. Be cautious for gut health and homeostasis of the body. That being said, there are some wonderful system support oils for internal use, and we will discuss some of them later in this section. Some people should not use oils internally due to a medication and/or health condition. Please note my disclaimer and always consult with your health professional prior to use if you are on medication and/or have a health condition.

Aren't all oils created equally? Most certainly not! Did you know...

- Oil can be labeled pure and be taken from a less powerful, less expensive, easier to source part of the plant. Where the quality of oil comes in for helping support the body systems is in its source with every plant being different. On some plants, it's the bud; others it's the leaf, and others might be the root. The point is, you want it from the most powerful part of the plant, not the cheapest and most available for the supplier to obtain.

- Oil can be obtained by the extraction method, which means a chemical is used to extract the essential oil. The oil can also be obtained through distillation, which means through using steam (by far more preferable).
- Oil can be labeled pure and distilled but distilled at higher heat in order to obtain the essential oil faster. More bottles of oil to market means more profit.

I admire and respect that Young Living:

- Slowly distills the oil to gently obtain the oil from the plant. Gentle distillation means less chance of damaging the chemical constituent of the plant with the end result being quality over profit.
- Has control of the growth process. It's vital for you to pick a carrot from your garden at its peak for optimum nutrition; the same applies for when to harvest a plant to extract its essential oil. Owning the farms controls harvest time.
- Uses essential oils as weed control and fertilizer; there are no chemicals/fertilizers or insecticides.
- Has integrity with decades of experience.
- These were all deciding factors in my choosing Young Living Essential oils seven years ago. I have never regretted that decision. When you add in testimonies of the hundreds of thousands of Young Living essential oils users feeling amazing body support, it

proves the ability and integrity of Young Living oils.

Safety Recommendations

Due to the potency of these gifts from nature, it's important to respect them. For your benefit, here are some safety tips.

1. If you are pregnant, nursing, taking medication, or have a medical condition, consult a health professional prior to use on all Young Living supplements and oils including oil blends.

2. Read and follow all label cautions and warnings.

3. Teach children that EOs are to be respected; keep out of reach of children and pets.

4. When using a new oil, always dilute to avoid skin sensitivity. It's also a good idea to conduct a patch test of diluted essential oil on the inner arm before using; discontinue use if skin gets irritated.

5. Never drop EOs directly into eyes or ears.

6. If you get an EO in your eye, do NOT use water to dilute as that will drive the EO in further. Instead, dilute immediately with a carrier oil such as a pure coconut, olive, avocado, or Young Livings V6 carrier oil.

7. If oil feels hot or irritating on your skin, do not use water. Instead, dilute it with carrier oil such as those listed above.

8. Some EOs are photosensitive, meaning you can burn or pigment skin if going in the sun after applying these oils. Consult an essential oils' reference guide book on photosensitivity if in doubt on whether the EO you want to use is photosensitive.

9. Use caution and avoid hot EOs with children and pets (e.g., clove, cinnamon, oregano). Check your essential oils' references for more

safety tips with children and pets.

10. If you add an EO to liquids, be sure not to use plastic since oils can erode the plastic thus putting chemicals in your water. Glass is my top choice for this type of use.

11. Avoid setting EOs directly on furniture or areas that can be damaged. EOs can damage the surface.

12. Young Living labels each bottle of Young Living essential oil with directions for how to use it; these directions vary based on your region. Please consult the product label for appropriate usage directions.

13. If you have sensitive skin, epilepsy, heart or kidney problems, or any serious medical condition, do not use essential oils unless advised by a physician or medical professional that it is safe.

For more complete safety tips and recommendations, consult a complete version reference guide for essential oils. I will provide links to several websites that sell reference books and brochures as well as glass bottles and jars for your home recipes, diffusers, and more.

Four-Pronged Approach

While it is important to support each and every one of the body systems, we will focus in this chapter on the body systems mentioned in this book: the digestive, endocrine, and nervous systems. This obviously does not mean we don't need to deal with the other systems, but if we first focus on one or two systems for offering support, we are best able to gauge our body response.

Each body system interacts with and supports the others. By supporting body *systems* rather than individual glands or organs, we take out some of the guesswork. If I provide my endocrine system with the oil blend called EndoFlex, I'm supporting the entire system. The body will choose how and where to use the constituents of that particular essential oil to maintain balance of the system. Our job is to offer the support; the body takes the support to utilize it where needed.

As a reminder on whole body health, we know oils cannot cure this or that malady. Knowing what you now know about leaky gut and insulin, do you think oils could ever have brought Karly's hormones into balance without approaching leaky gut and balancing insulin levels through stress removal, diet, and toxins removal? No, they could not. What cures is the human body. And the human body can only do this when it is given the tools to do so. What are these tools? We have discussed them extensively in the main part of this book. Whole foods. Chemical-free foods. Nurturing foods. Nutritious foods. A more relaxed mind and body. We use these things to bring the body above the wellness line then offer support to the body systems through EOs and supplements. Only using oils would be a one-pronged approach. We have to look at least four prongs to our health program:

1. Diet
2. Removing toxins/chemicals
3. Stress relief/support
4. Support and soothe body systems (including digestive system) with supplements and essential oils!

This is the four-pronged approach. Guess what else has four prongs? Your fork! There will be no supplement, powder, or oil that will help your body if the diet is not good. Almost to a person, every woman with hormone issues admits to strong sugar cravings and intake when I talk to her. We can support already healthy insulin levels with EOs (I have my favorites for this), but if the sugar intake continues, there will continue to be health issues. Sugar decimates gut and liver health; thus, it decimates hormone balance. There is no way around this cycle of damage. So pay attention to what's on that fork (or spoon) every single time it enters your mouth.

When we clean up our diet, our lifestyle, and ease our stress, we have a body that will kick into high gear to achieve balance (homeostasis). As our body reaches homeostasis and achieves wellness, it can greatly benefit from the support of EOs so that the body systems can maintain that proper function. Supporting is where EOs come into play. EOs have been used since Biblical times and are used by people all over the world. EO users include chiropractors, young mothers and grandmothers, pharmacists, nurses and doctors, construction workers, and children; literally millions of people have brought EOs into their home in an effort to reduce toxins and support their body systems.

You can use EOs as your doorway into the world of supporting your body with natural means. They can uplift spirits. They can provide digestive and liver support. They can uplift mood through their aromatic compounds. They can possibly even bring hope where once there was none (as in our case). When we use EOs to support a positive attitude and lifestyle, we no longer want or need the toxins in food and products that used to be a big part of our life.

I am going to list suggested Young Living products for supporting the digestive, endocrine, and nervous systems. Some books on body systems will separate the endocrine and reproductive systems, but I will combine the two; endocrine system support products will include the reproductive system.

Young Living has a long list of amazing single oils and oil blends for support of the nervous system. Even though I will be listing products for this system, I'm not going into the variety of areas we could support the nervous system such as focus. Rather, I'm going to list those that deal with areas most females need daily that we have covered in the main part of the book: relaxing and comforting the nervous system. Our goal here is to slow down those racing thoughts to help maintain and support healthy cortisol levels since it's a huge influence on our endocrine/hormone system.

After listing these systems and support products, I will list products Karly and I use daily as an example of how we have incorporated this support into our lives. I will follow that information with a more detailed description for each of these products. However, I will skip the standard EO information for each oil and their individual uses from the Young Living website. That would get far too expansive and lose focus on why we are here: to find ways to support our endocrine/hormone, digestive, and nervous systems. I will list why we like the particular oil in our daily protocol as well as how we use it. For full discussions on all the EOs in Young Livings lineup, safety precautions, and uses, visit the Young Living website or look into a good reference book on essential oils. Many can be located in the links I will provide for EO materials.

Keep in mind that we are all snowflakes—alike but very different. Our favorite daily oils and how we use them may not be what is your top choice or fit your particular situation. You may need support in an entirely different area such as cardiovascular or excretory systems. I list our use only as examples of how to incorporate these natural products into your life with the understanding you should research to see which of these you might want to try as well as safety recommendations. Ease into any new supplement and product you use; be attentive to body response and adjust accordingly. Now let's get to work because we have much to discuss regarding essential oils and body support!

Chapter Twenty-Two: How to Use Essential Oils

A common question is "How do I use these oils?" While I like to look at four main ways, a person can pretty much, if in doubt, slightly dilute an EO with a carrier oil (e.g., coconut, almond, olive oil) and apply topically. You can apply topically to an area of concern, such as an aching muscle, or you can apply to the wrists for absorption through the thin skin into the bloodstream to have the constituents of the oil carried throughout the body. How to use them is not a rigid protocol. There are some possible ways one EO may serve its purpose better, but applying it topically will still get it into your body so you won't really go wrong with this use. Here are the ways we commonly use EOs.

Topical

Dilute with carrier oil (not canola or corn oil) and apply. With topical application, we should have the constituents of the oil circulated throughout the body within about twenty minutes. Apply to the area of concern, or you can also apply to the VitaFlex point on the bottom of your foot. Some of our largest pores are on the bottom of our feet to help with absorption into the body. Plus, due to thicker skin, our feet are prone to less skin sensitization making them a safer place to begin using oils. Another good reason for the feet? If it's not your favorite smelling oil or you are going to be in a confined area where the aroma might bother others, you can apply, let it absorb, cover with a bit of carrier oil, and put your socks and/or shoes on where the smell can remain. This is better than wrists or neck where you will be wearing the potent EO smell throughout the day. If it's a beautiful smell, go for it on the body, but if it's not a pretty smell, try the feet. Your office neighbor or church pew partner will thank you. It's important to remember, the scent of oil can be overpowering to a non-user, even if we love the smell. We really don't want to turn someone off to the beauty of EOs by overwhelming his or her senses. It's like sitting next to someone with a strong perfume. To them, it's a beautiful smell, but to us, it may be annoying. So, please respect others when using your oils.

Inhalation

The sense of smell is the most powerful way to access our emotions through the amygdala—our emotional control center. Even though the amygdala is enclosed within the highly protective blood-brain barrier, EO's lipids are allowed to permeate this membrane to access our emotional control center. Isn't that more than just a little amazing? Inhalation of EOs is the fastest (approximately twenty-two seconds) and most powerful way to deliver the molecularly minuscule constituents of an EO into the nervous system and eventually the entire body. The capillary-rich, mucosal nasal membranes make them an excellent vehicle for absorption of the constituents in each EO. While inhalation provides the fastest delivery, the effect also dissipates the fastest. Due to the potential for a powerful effect, inhalation for the elderly and children may be a bit much; you may want to consider diffusing or using on their feet instead.

Diffusing

This method is gentler than inhalation but an effective way to deliver the oils constituents through the nasal membranes to the amygdala and throughout

350

the body. This is a great way to gently use them for baby, children, and ourselves at bedtime to absorb while we are sleeping. I like this method for children and elderly—daytime or night, it helps with slower and gentler absorption. Always introduce during the day the first few times of use so you can absorb effects.

Internal

This can be done through a drop or two of EO in a capsule, glass of water, milk, or in food. Only use Young Livings Vitality™ line for approved internal use.

Let's move on to look at how can we use EOs to support the three body systems we are addressing in this book: the nervous, digestive, and endocrine systems.

Supporting the Nervous System

Why begin with the nervous system? Because our number one area we must address before all else is support for our nervous system since any reaction in the nervous system sends out a complicated array of messages to every single control center—muscles, nerves, fibers, hormone-secreting glands—of our body. Tense muscles? Blame the nervous system. Heart beating out of your chest? Look to the nervous system. Sad and dreary? Yeah...that's the nervous system once again.

Think of what happens when we get wired or uptight: the message goes out. We tense our shoulders, our throat, and other areas that ultimately restrict proper blood flow. If we don't have proper blood flow, we interfere with support the muscular and skeletal areas preventing in coming to balance in that area. The same applies to all body systems; the messages sent from our nervous system ultimately affect these systems to either support or interfere with our daily functions. Thus, we begin with the nervous system—the big kahuna of all body systems. While dealing with life situations that interfere with normal moods we can utilize exercise, breathing EFT, and we can also offer the soothing aroma of EOs to support these methods. The beauty of this is that the aromatic constituents in some EOs have the ability to absorb through nasal membranes to be delivered to the amygdala—your emotional control center—of the nervous system to help soothe and balance.

Supporting Moods

So let's discuss how we can support healthy moods. A typical day may be we have a desk piled high with work. We know we have children to pick up, get home, feed, and then head to school conferences. After that, children need homework done, baths, and put to bed. I'll admit this takes me back to the days when my kids were young. My stress levels go up just writing this! Let's get back to you sitting at work knowing all this is ahead of you along with your file folders of work piled high. What happens? Your brain starts going in circles. The amygdala sends out the fight-or-flight signals, and the adrenals start kicking out cortisol in mass quantities. Meanwhile, you are bottling things up because, honestly, what else can you do? Well, I suggest get up from your desk, take a quick walk down the hallways to release some of that tension, then back to the desk and inhale some frankincense or lavender while using your 4-7-8 breathing technique. The slow, deep breaths along with the constituents in the EO—absorbing into the nasal membranes, which then deliver the constituents in the oil to the amygdala—are a great way to help settle down and unwind while the deep breaths help us deal with how we react to the stress. We didn't remove the stressors, but we did control our response. Your adrenals, liver, and ultimately, your hormone balance will all appreciate this way of dealing with life rather than holding things in.

We have discussed different ways to reduce stress: exercise, prayer, meditation, proper diet, breathing techniques as well as acupuncture, massage, and chiropractic. Each of these can be enhanced with the addition of the calming aroma of essential oils to support your nervous system when life gets a little crazy. In addition, inhaling, diffusing, and applying EOs topically can support your body's ability to dissipate negative emotions. Let's look at some examples of how to use EOs in conjunction with our relaxation techniques to assist in dealing with day-to-day problems

1. **We can inhale an essential oil while we use our 4-7-8 breathing technique.** This is one of my favorite ways to bring my wired brain down several notches to a more level state, especially at bedtime. As discussed, this breathing technique is excellent for calming and dealing with stress. Now, let's include the soothing aroma of an oil like lavender, bergamot, or any number of oils I will list under nervous system support. The breathing technique combined with the soothing aroma of an EO can help us unwind at the end of a busy day.

2. **We can inhale or diffuse an EO while practicing meditation.** According to 2013 abstract from the Department of Psychiatry at Srinakharinwirot University, "Mindfulness meditation lowers the cortisol levels in the blood suggesting that it can lower stress." Meditation is powerful for stress reduction while the soothing or uplifting scent of an EO contributes to a more beneficial meditation session, which ultimately allows meditation to have an impact on lowering cortisol levels in a powerful way.

3. **We can use an EO to enhance an exercise session** by diffusing, inhaling YL peppermint oil, or using a drop or two of the Vitality™ Oil in our water prior to our workout. Harvard Health Publications' 2011 article "Exercising to Relax" claims "exercise reduces levels of the body's stress hormones, such as adrenaline and cortisol." Adding in the uplifting benefits of peppermint oil (or many other EO possibilities), which may support exercise performance to help you have a great workout, is an excellent idea. Remember our caveat on exercise; excessive endurance exercise/hard cardio workouts only increase the stress on the adrenals and body, which will elevate cortisol. Elevating cortisol is a surefire way to retain those extra pounds you were hoping to lose. Keep it simple but effective when it comes to exercise and avoiding elevated cortisol.

The same principle of using EOs applies to any of our stress-reducing practices such as prayer, yoga, chiropractic, acupuncture, Reiki, or massage. Virtually any relaxing, stress-reducing techniques can help us but when you add the support from the soothing, uplifting effect of an EO, you just ramped up to support that benefit exponentially.

Since inhalation is a great way to use EOs for fast and effective action while topical application will allow for absorption into the body for longer lasting benefit, I like the one-two punch provided by doing the following: Use inhalation of a soothing or empowering EO aroma for a fast, effective way to uplift or ease loss of control. Knowing the response will dissipate faster than topical, I follow up with topical application, which will have slower immediate effect but will last longer than inhalation.

Amid all this discussion in the main part of this book on toxins, sugars, and elevated cortisol, let's remember how they interfere with balanced hormone production. Laughter and enjoyment of life are an important part of helping the body deal with life's daily struggles. We need to include the important benefit of living fully, with a positive focus to help our mental state and body health. EOs are an excellent way to help to uplift and energize a mental attitude. Feeling down? Inhale or diffuse some bergamot or lavender or peppermint or lemon or...(you get the idea).

How EOs Support

What are some great EOs to support the nervous system? YL has a wide array of EOs, and those listed below are just some that we can use. You may find one that contributes to your well-being that isn't even on this list, and that's great. The important thing is to know there are many options and techniques available. The best way to find your favorite combo is to actually use them. Far too many people get their oils, set them on a closet shelf, and that's the last they see of them. Take them out, apply them, inhale them, diffuse them. Whatever you do, use your EOs. There is no absolute right or wrong way except not to use them at all. I consider that a very wrong way.

Good ways to use your oils for nervous system support are to inhale, diffuse, dilute slightly, and apply topically at the base of the skull/top of neck in back, over the liver area, or on the bottom of each big toe—the VitaFlex points for the brain. Here are some common favorites for support. While there are many to choose from, I am narrowing it down to give you some focus for ideas of where to begin. I will indicate some of these as personal favorites by placing a double asterisk (**) next to those I feel should be in every household for everyday use. Give one or each of them a try and, if you like the effect, circle the oil on the next page to help you track which ones are most beneficial to you.

Nervous System Support (**Personal Favorites)

Single Oils	Oil Blends	Supplements
Lavender**	Joy™**	MindWise™
Frankincense**	Release™**	Ningxia Red®**
Peppermint**	Stress Away™**	Mineral Essence™**
Balsam Fir	Peace & Calming™**	OmegaGize3®**
Melissa	Clarity™	
Bergamot	Brain Power™	
Clary Sage	Humility™**	
German Chamomile	Peace & Calming II™	
Lemon**	Harmony™	
Vetiver	Oola Fun™	
Cedarwood	Gratitude™	
Ylang Ylang**	Gentle Baby™	

Ningxia Red offers whole body support so it really could be listed under any of the body systems. I am including it under nervous system health support products, however, it's not only the nervous system but every single body system that can be supported with Ningxia Red.

Supporting the Digestive System

Let's move on to our next body system to support, the digestive system. We know how important this system is to our entire body health. It has the potential to avoid or contribute to inflammation, depending on the health of our gut lining. Even though the liver is part of the digestive system, it's highly influential to our hormone balance, which is technically related to endocrine system as well. This demonstrates the eventual interplay between systems where, what happens in one, affects others. The liver is a key player in metabolizing and synthesizing our estrogens (good and bad estrogens). We need to support proper liver health, our clearing-house of toxins. When the liver is overloaded, it can't clear toxins. This affects its ability to help us maintain estrogen balance, which can ultimately contribute to estrogen dominance and progesterone deficiency. We don't want that to happen, otherwise, female hormone conditions make their appearance. (Remember Xeno taking over the body?) Good liver health, even though it is part of our digestive system, is vital to hormone regulation and overall health.

In order for us to keep putting one foot in front of the other, we need food to provide energy to help our body repair, reproduce, and grow. The digestion system is designed to perform these functions. Its purpose is to extract the essence from the food that we eat and discard the indigestible part as waste. The best way to help the digestive system perform correctly? Through proper support!

On the next page are *some* digestive system oils and supplements from Young Living. I will discuss these in more detail after listing the recommended oils and products for both the digestive and endocrine systems. Once again, there are a plethora of options. However, some of these are musts, in my opinion.

Digestive System Support (**Personal Favorites)

Single Oils

Peppermint

Peppermint Vitality™**

Ginger Vitality™

Fennel

Lemon Vitality™**

Lemongrass Vitality™

Coriander

Dill Vitality™

Black Pepper Vitality™

Copaiba Vitality™**

Oil Blends

DiGize™**

Aroma Ease™

Liver Support

GLF™

JuvaFlex®**

Juva Cleanse™

JuvaTone®**

Juva Power®

Supplements

ICP™

ComforTone®**

Digest & Cleanse**

AlkaLime®

Digestive Enzymes

Essentialzyme™**

Essentialzyme-4™**

Allerzyme™

DeToxyme™**

Endocrine System (Hormone) Support (**Personal Favorites)

Single Oils	Oil Blends	Supplements / Personal Care
Ocotea**	Dragon Time™**	Progessence Plus™**
Lavender**	Sclaressence™**	Prenolone+™
Clary Sage	EndoFlex™ & EndoFlex Vitality™**	Thyromin™**
Fennel	Shutran™**	CortiStop™
Geranium	Mister™	EndoGize™
Idaho Blue Spruce**		Prostate Health™** (Men)
Goldenrod		

Phytoestrogens

What about the constituent known as phytoestrogens found in some plants from which EOs are distilled? In general, phytoestrogens are weaker than the natural estrogen hormones (such as estradiol) found in humans and animals or the very potent synthetic estrogens used in birth control pills and other drugs, according to *Journal of Chromatography's* 2002 article "Assessing estrogenic activity of phytochemicals using transcriptional activation and immature mouse uterotrophic responses."

There are two schools of thought on this topic. Some think phytoestrogens cause health issues while others believe they offer support to the body. Remember, "Phyto" estrogens from a plant are vastly different than "Xeno" estrogens, which are powerful hormone disruptors caused from chemicals in our environment. Think of your hormones as messengers sent to deliver the mail. They knock on many doors, but none open until the cell (address) waiting for that mail. Many UPS and FedEx messengers (other chemical constituents) have traveled past that same door but didn't stop to drop off their hormone chemical because the delivery (chemical) did not have that cell door's address. When the chemical constituent and the cell needing it match, the delivery is made because the key fit that one particular door or cell receptor.

Phytoestrogens are considered to offer their constituent (mail) to the estrogen cell receptor sites. Remember, if the mail isn't supposed to be delivered to that address, the door won't open. If the constituent (phytoestrogen) is wanted, the cell accepts the delivery. If the constituent is not wanted or does not fit, it is not accepted and moves on to be easily excreted from the body, as it is a natural substance easily broken down and eliminated.

Phytoestrogens are very weak compared to our own natural estrogen according to nutrition expert Rachel Beller. Beller as noted in the Beller Nutritional Institute explained that while phytoestrogens are similar to human estrogens, their effect on human estrogen levels has not been well researched because plant estrogens are 1,000 times weaker than the estrogen produced in our bodies.

Synthetic hormones (including birth control pills) contain constituents created in a lab that stick or attach to the cell receptors whether the receptors want the mail delivered or not. Xenoestrogens, the powerful estrogen mimickers (10-100 times more powerful than our natural estrogen), are created from chemicals or toxins introduced to our body through food and personal care products. They set up residence, binding to cell receptors while being difficult to break down and eliminate.

Dr. John R. Lee, author of the book *The Breakthrough Book on Natural Hormone Balance* writes, "...phytoestrogens [are] weakly active plant estrogens that occupy cell receptors that, by competition, block out the more toxic xenoestrogens" in *What Your Doctor May Not Tell You About Menopause.* This school of thought on phytoestrogens is that they compete for the cell receptor to help block the absorption of the powerful, disrupting xenoestrogens. Think of it as this room is taken, keep on moving. This, to me, is powerful. With all the xenoestrogens in our environment and, with so much estrogen dominance, we need to consider ways to help our bodies handle these chemicals.

Thus, we have major differences between natural phytoestrogens versus synthetic hormones (including birth control pills) and hormone mimickers, xenoestrogens.

Phytoestrogens = Up to 1,000 times weaker than our natural estrogen. Offered to the cell receptor and absorbed if the key is a fit to the cell receptor door. A tap on the cell door.

Synthetic hormones/Xenoestrogens = 10-100 times more powerful than our natural estrogen. Due to their chemical makeup and power, they tell the cell it's coming in rather than asking. A rap on the cell door.

Which would you rather have in your body? A mild phytoestrogen occupying the cell receptor to allow support for proper function (and since the receptor is occupied, it leaves no room for the xenoestrogens) or a powerful, disrupting, chemically created xenoestrogen taking up residence and in no hurry to depart the body? By allowing the phytoestrogen to occupy the cell receptor, Dr. Lee is suggesting the xenoestrogen cannot occupy the receptor. That's pretty impressive.

There's also a great deal of debate surrounding phytoestrogens due to articles listing bad effects. Most of these articles are related to the isoflavones in soy. Non-GMO fermented soy has helped Asian women sail through life tremendously better than American women for centuries until GMOs entered the picture as well as leaving out the fermentation process with unfermented soy. The problem very likely isn't the isoflavones with phytoestrogens in soy but the GMO soy, which is most soy on the market today. Women, as well as men, should avoid soy just to be on the safe side.

There are a tremendous number of articles on the topic of phytoestrogens. I encourage you to research (and eliminate those citing results/testing involving soy for the reason listed above) so you can make an informed decision whether you should avoid EOs with phytoestrogens. Also, be sure you give fair measure to scientifically backed natural health sites as much as you do western-based medicine sites that weigh in the favor of pharmaceuticals.

Like everything we use in and on our bodies, it's good to avoid overuse. More is not always better, and caution is better than overindulgence. As mentioned earlier, EOs are powerful and have the potential for both benefit or harm depending on your use. Harm with an oil is unlikely if you research usage and avoid overuse. We do not need ten drops of oil in a capsule (as I have seen recommended on some sites). We ease into use of each new oil or product. We offer small amounts. We gauge responses and adjust accordingly. It's also good to take a day off about once a week to give your body filters a rest so they can regenerate and recuperate. Rest is good for us, and it's good for our body organs and systems.

Chapter Twenty-Three: Daily Essential Oils

I am including Young Living supplements as well as essential oils. When I first started using Young Living essential oils, I was aware they had supplements but had no interest in using them. My thought was, "What does an essential oil company know about supplements? There are plenty of companies that produce only supplements so they would be specialists and likely have better supplements." My mind slowly changed as I read more and more about Young Living supplements. Why? Two reasons.

They contain essential oils—a huge benefit. It's as much about absorption as it is about the quantity of nutrients in the supplement. Some brands list a large percent of nutrients in their supplement. Often this is so they can be sure you absorb at least the minimum amount needed for benefit. The downside of this is your liver and kidneys are stuck filtering out the excess. When you use multiple supplements per day and do this day after day, your already overworked organs have an extra, unnecessary burden. Essential oils aid in the absorption of your nutrients so fewer nutrients are needed for the same effect.

According to the April 2016 edition of *Natural Awakenings,* "Recent clinical experience has discovered a huge difference in greens without the addition of essential oils versus the addition of essential oils." Thus, you will note on most of YL's supplements, the levels of ingredients aren't usually large amounts—which is good news to your liver and kidneys.

Young Living has an impeccable history and reputation for avoiding fillers and cheap ingredients in their supplements. Fillers are the type of things build up and cause stress on our already overworked body filters.

I have listed some EOs and supplements normally used for support to the body systems we are discussing in this book. For those unfamiliar with EOs, I thought it might be beneficial to go through my daily oils, which turns out to be pretty much the same as my daughter's. My age is fifty-nine years old, and Karly is twenty-eight years old. This gives two different age groups for females yet the basics of nervous, digestive, endocrine systems support are almost the same for each of us. This is not an accident. My school of thought with every single female (and male) remains: support the foundation of what the body needs with slight variances for our age and adjust for individual situations after the foundation is supported. There are really only two areas we vary from each other in our daily protocol. I will note those products that are unique to my protocol versus Karly's as I discuss them in the next section.

By giving you the list of EOs we use, I am not necessarily saying our usage would be your protocol, but rather, I am wanting you to get an idea how an average oils user might incorporate them into their lives. Let's take a look...*

Our Daily Basics

Remember to have a day of rest about once per week.

Oils	Supplements
Ocotea Oil	MultiGreens™
JuvaFlex Blend	Super B™
Lemon Vitality™ Oil	Ningxia Red™
DragonTime™ (*Karly only)	OmegaGize ™ (fish oil)
Sclaressence™ (*Teri only)	Life 5™ (probiotics)
EndoFlex™	Essentialzyme™ (digestive enzymes)
Peppermint & Peppermint Vitality™	Thyromin
Vitality™	
DiGize™ Oil Blend	
StressAway™	
Lavender & Lavender Vitality™	
Progessence Plus™ *	
Copaiba Vitality™	

(*Teri only on PP at this time. Karly will use this to maintain wellness once she attains a wellness level of progesterone from her bioidentical progesterone troche.)

These products are our favorite products used daily other than our day of rest. With over 140 single oils and oil blends in Young Living's repertoire, we obviously cannot discuss all of them. Therefore, I will discuss why we use the ones above as well as list several other favorites after discussing the hows and whys of our favorites. That should keep you busy! Let's take a look at one of our top oils.

Ocotea Oil

Yes, this is our #1. That doesn't mean it should be yours although you may want to give it some consideration. Why? From the cinnamon family, Ocotea helps aid the body's natural response to irritation and injury and may support healthy digestion including satiety. When we consider the extreme stress—both emotionally and physically—our bodies are subjected to, my experience with Ocotea for supporting my body's response to irritation has been excellent. What's my #1 eating concern for all men and women today? Sugar intake. What will the body do with high sugar intake? Secrete insulin in large amounts to deal with that sugar. What organ gets irritated day after day due to this? Our pancreas. Therefore, since Ocotea has the potential to aid and support in the body's response to irritation and the pancreas is vital to hormone balance. For supporting a healthy pancreas, I greatly favor this oil. What could be more important than supporting the organ that secretes our master hormone, insulin? Ocotea is also rich in the constituent alpha humulene; compliance keeps me from listing the benefits of this great constituent, but I encourage you to do a web search and read up on it.

How to Use

Approved usage is topical. I apply two drops of Ocotea neat or undiluted (slightly dilute if you haven't used it before in case of skin irritation) over my pancreas morning and night. In addition, YL's Blend Slique Essence (for support of healthy weight-management goals) contains Ocotea (as well as citrus oils with spearmint). This is approved for internal use so, if I want to include Ocotea in my daily protocol *internally, I* turn to Slique Essence™. Either way, both Karly and I make sure to use Ocotea oil every day.

Ningxia Red Drink

Often we are concerned (and confused) with where to start, as each of us has different systems (and sometimes a multitude of systems) we want to address. Ningxia Red Drink rates right at the top for me for the beauty of how many ways it supports overall wellness. Before we shotgun approach things by trying to target different systems, organs, and glands, we can support the overall foundation of the body by drinking one ounce of Ningxia morning and afternoon. (Avoid evening, as Ningxia tends to energize us.) Supporting the foundation may help support the body enough that other areas in need may now be doing just fine, possibly making the EOs and supplements you were going to use in those areas unnecessary.

By consuming the multitude of vitamins, nutrients, minerals, and antioxidants in Ningxia that also includes four essential oils, we have a powerhouse of support. It is the only drink in the world (to my knowledge) loaded with these types of nutrients *and* essential oils to help the cells absorb those nutrients and antioxidants. Don't skim over the word antioxidants. These are our anti-rusting constituents and are essential to helping the body maintain wellness. At my age, avoiding "rusting" is super important. Ningxia

367

was one of the last things I added to my daily protocol. I hadn't given it much consideration since I didn't want to spend the money. As I observed the results of some of my friends and YL members, it became clear I needed to re-think my attitude and do more research. That's exactly what I did, which has led me to four years of continual use.

I'll keep it short and sweet, but I think it's important to list the ingredients in this drink so you can visualize just how many excellent constituents it contains.

- Orange, Yuzu, Lemon, and Tangerine essential oils in NingXia Red contain d-limonene, which is a powerful wellness-promoting constituent. (Research D-Limonene, a constituent in many of the citrus oils.)

- When compared to other antioxidant drinks on the market, Independent test from Brunswick Laboratories surmised that **NingXia Red**® contains the highest amount of antioxidants of any drink on the market.

- NingXia Red is free of high fructose sweeteners or added sugar; it does contain added Stevia for taste.

- Ningxia contains wolfberries and exotic fruits concentrate (not juice) such as blueberry, cherry, aronia, pomegranate, and plum.

- Ningxia has valuable minerals, amino acids, and antioxidants.

- When we look to provide ourselves with a healthy alternative to sugary drinks, Ningxia is a great choice. There are even recipes for popsicles and gummy bears. (If anyone makes these, feel free to send me a bag!)

EndoFlex™ Oil Blend or EndoFlex Vitality™ Blend

Next up on my list of favorites is the EndoFlex™ Blend. We have mentioned our endocrine system as being the control center of our hormone secretion. Think of how many important glands and organs are in this system; the thyroid, adrenals, pancreas, and ovaries are only a partial list. Are there any of those you feel don't need support? If so, think again... our lifestyles put constant stress on the entire system. Therefore, we might avoid the shotgun approach of trying to target multiple glands with multiple oils or supplements by using one blend to support one very important system: ENDOFlex™ blend for our ENDOcrine system. Use this oil blend on a regular basis as one of your mainstays—you might avoid purchasing a bunch of single oils.

This great blend is comprised of a base of sesame seed oil, spearmint, sage, myrtle, nutmeg, and German chamomile. The properties of these oils may offer a variety of support. With all the stressors in our lives, the thyroid is one of the first to try and compensate when other systems are failing to keep up with their balancing act, so supporting response to irritation is a big plus. This is the reason I like topical application over the thyroid. When you look at the power of combining the constituents in these oils, you have to admire Young Livings founder and owner of Young Living, Gary Young (which I do constantly) for his amazing wisdom on this blend.

How to Use

I apply one to two drops of EndoFlex™ Blend topically over my thyroid (front of neck, halfway down, rub on each side of windpipe) and adrenals (located mid-back on top the kidneys) morning and afternoon. Avoid EndoFlex™ blend near bedtime, as some of the oils in this blend can energize—a great thing during the day but not so great at bedtime.

If I want to take it internally, I substitute EndoFlex Vitality™ Blend for EndoFlex™ topical application. Remember they are both made up of the same single oils but are only labeled differently due to usage—topical versus internal. If I use EndoFlex Vitality™, I either put 1-2 drops on my finger and swipe inside my cheek or I place 1-2 drops under the tongue and hold for about one minute for absorption. I would do this morning and afternoon just like the topical EndoFlex™ Blend. Either type of use should offer support. If you use it topically for a few weeks and don't feel you are getting support, try internal with EndoFlex™ Vitality Blend.

SclarEssence™ Oil Blend

Once I hit the age of fifty, this blend became one of my "can't live without" oils. It was created for support of healthy female hormones and a healthy glandular system. Remember our endocrine system is comprised of multiple glands. If you are a younger lady, this blend is still great for support for you although many younger women (including my daughter) like DragonTime™ Blend a tad more, which we will discuss next. Not only did adding this blend to my daily protocol help support mood, it also was also great for that healthy glandular support and wellness so I don't have to worry about a body temperature meltdown 10-12 times per day like many women my age.

What are the oils in this blend? A single oil containing a constituent called sclareol (hence the name of this blend) has been used for centuries by women of all ages for support of normal, healthy attitude regardless what day of the month it might be. It also contains peppermint oil, which is great for its cooling effect and liver support. Fennel is another great oil in this blend that was used all the way back in ancient times when it was used by Egyptian women for support of healthy female hormone balance. In addition, this blend contains sage lavender or Spanish sage oil, which can contribute to emotional balancing and relaxation.

So, we have the soothing effects as well as liver support of peppermint, support of healthy female hormones in fennel, and clary sage with the calming action of sage lavender. This is exactly why this blend is near the top of my list. I like to pair Sclaressence™ with Progessence Plus™, the Yin and Yang (opposing but complementary) of support for overall wellness, something all females can use as they get older and life throws curveballs at us!

If you have issues with your endocrine system balance, please consult with your health professional for testing and information regarding bioidentical hormone support. If you are seeking support of healthy balance, consider Sclaressence™ (with Progessence Plus). Some of the oils in this blend contain the natural phytoestrogens oils we discussed earlier. If this is a concern for you, refer to the previous chapter as a review of this topic and consult with your health professional with any questions or concerns.

How to Use

Approved use for Sclaressence™ is topical. You can apply to your ankles, both inside and outside of ankle right above the anklebone. I start with 2-3 drops morning and evening but depending on how much support you want, you can adjust accordingly. Since this blend is great for healthy mood support, many women like to use this according to their cycle if they still have a period; they don't use for roughly seven days and then re-start for the next twenty-one days at the end of their cycle. If you no longer have period, I still use it for about twenty-one days and then take a seven-day rest. Use however it makes you feel best supported.

371

Dragon Time™ Oil Blend

As I mentioned above, you can interchange Sclaressence™ and Dragon Time™ as they have an overlap of oils. However, if both blends were readily available to me and I still had a monthly period, I would lean toward Dragon Time. Both blends have clary sage and fennel for support of healthy female cycles. Dragon Time™ blend does not have peppermint and sage like Sclaressence™, but it does have several oils that Sclaressence™ does not such as jasmine, lavender, marjoram, and yarrow. Therefore, this blend is aiming a little more at supporting a normal emotional state and occasional nervous tension of young ladies with fluctuating cycles and moods combined with the qualities of clary sage and fennel for support of female balance. Marjoram also eases muscle tension (the abdomen has lots of muscles!). The aroma of Dragon Time™ is designed to invite positive emotions for women, especially during their monthly cycle.

If you have issues with your endocrine system balance, please consult with your health professional for testing and information regarding bioidentical hormone support. If you are seeking support of healthy balance, consider Dragon Time™ (with Progessence Plus™).

How to Use

Approved use for Dragon Time™ is topical. You can apply to your ankles, both inside and outside of ankle right above the anklebone, over the ovaries, and/or on the wrists. You can start with 2-3 drops morning and evening, but depending on how much support you want, you can adjust accordingly. If you are having a bad day, use more and more often. Many women like to use this according to their cycle with no use during their period and then restarting for the next twenty-one days at the end of their period.

It's a good idea to pair Dragon Time ™ Blend with Progessence Plus™, the Yin and Yang (opposing but complementary) of support for overall wellness plus the aroma helps support mood to help you be nicer to your spouse. (They call it Dragon Time for a reason!) Some of the oils in this blend contain the natural phytoestrogens we discussed earlier. Refer to the previous chapter as a review of this topic and consult with your health professional with any questions or concerns.

Progessence Plus Serum™ Oil

Progessence Plus Serum™ is one of the biggest blessings Young Living (along with Dr. Dan Purser) has ever delivered. This serum is made with essential oils and wild yam extract designed to support overall women's wellness and harmonizing normal cycles. It is a gentle, soothing serum and can be used by both younger and older women. This is a great one to use near bedtime to let go of the day's problems and promote relaxation.

Check out the excellent combination of oils in this one: frankincense, bergamot, cedarwood, copaiba, peppermint, clove, rosewood, and the ingredients of USP Progesterone derived from wild yam root (Vitamin E-Caprylic/capric triglyceride). This is a combination of calming, uplifting, soothing oils for physical as well as emotional well-being. In this topsy-turvy world where we feel like everyone and everything demands our attention, Progessence Plus™ gives *us* the constituents we need for ourselves—both as a female and as an individual wanting to maintain and support our balance.

Remember, if you have issues with your endocrine system balance, please consult with your health professional for testing and information regarding progesterone or pregnenolone troches/capsules. If you want support for balance of healthy levels, consider Progessence Plus (with either Sclaressence™ or Dragon Time™).

How to Use

Something very awesome about this blend is how easy it is to use. As mentioned, I like to use it (especially the first few times) near bedtime. It truly may help us unwind to the point we want to slide into our cozy bed. For this reason, you don't want to use it first thing in the morning, at least when you first introduce it to your body. As they adjust, many women use it both morning and night. Its best absorption comes from applying to areas of the skin that are thin such as sides of the neck, wrists, inside upper thighs, forearms, etc. Although skin irritation is uncommon, because it contains peppermint (a "hotter" oil), you may need to alternate where you use it to avoid skin irritation. If no irritation, feel free to use where is most comfortable for you. I use 2-3 drops morning and night but if you are having the type of day where being a female is just no fun, you can always use more of it and more often.

Keep out of reach of children. If you're pregnant, nursing, taking medication, or if you have a medical condition, consult a healthcare practitioner prior to use. Do not use in conjunction with contraceptives containing progesterone.

Here's a note from Young Living regarding California's Proposition 65 warnings, which are legally required to be on our Progessence Plus product: Proposition 65 requires that products sold in California which carry any ingredients deemed to the California legislature to be hazardous to health must carry the warning you see on our label. In the case of Progessence

Plus, California requires the warning on all progesterone-containing products. However, California law does not distinguish between the synthetic medroxyprogesterone, which is the cause of California's concern, and the natural progesterone, which we derive from yams and which are widely used in the health industry. Both are generically referred to as "progesterone," which is the ingredient name in California's list. If you would like further information on this topic, we recommend you contact your healthcare professional for further information.

To clarify the above note, California requires a warning on *all* progesterone-type products regardless of being synthetic or natural. We have discussed the risks of synthetic progesterone in capsules and birth control pills earlier in this book. With studies showing the risks of these synthetics, California is doing a good thing warning women but "not so good" by not distinguishing natural/bioidentical from synthetic.

Copaiba Vitality™ Oil

From the Amazon region, this oil has traditionally been used to support the body's natural response to irritation and support healthy digestion. It has the highest content of beta-caryophyllene (by far) of all the essential oils. You may want to research and study the benefits of the constituent beta-caryophyllene. I use two drops every day in a capsule both for the irritation-response support as well as healthy digestion support.

Peppermint & Peppermint Vitality™ Oil

I will discuss both labels of Young Living's peppermint oil. Remember that the standard labeled peppermint oil with Young Living is the same oil, only approved for topical, diffusing, or inhalation use—not internal. While

Peppermint Vitality™ Oil is approved for internal use, not topical. They are the same oil with different labels and instructions on approved uses.

As a dietary aid, Peppermint Vitality™ rates right near the top as a must-have in our family. I like to use a drop or two after every meal for two reasons: it freshens my breath and aids in healthy digestion. You could add a drop or two to your water and drink it. Make sure it's only a small amount of water as it's not a good idea to drink a lot of fluid prior to/with or right after a meal.

Actually, this same use is what I do just prior to an exercise workout as well. Although I'm not an intense exerciser (which is good due to cortisol levels), I find it tough some days to motivate myself. The little bit I do for exercise isn't much—some hand weights, push-ups, and stretches—and yet there are still a number of days I come close to convincing myself it's fine to skip a day. Those are the days I want my Peppermint Vitality™ Oil. I use a few drops and get to work. It has an uplifting, energizing effect, which increases my time (and enjoyment) of working out. Maybe your exercise is an easy walk. That's OK. Use your oil, and you may find you pick up the pace a tad or walk longer than usual. Even better, if you walk far and your muscles are aching, use peppermint oil in a little olive or coconut oil and rub on the area for soothing comfort.

Another benefit to me, a woman over fifty, is for those times when you have too much coffee and your bladder informs you that you "gotta go, gotta go!" It doesn't leave much room for argument such as "I need to wait until the next gas station or until break time of this event I'm attending." Peppermint is a fun oil in that it contains the constituent methone to help create the aroma, which can energize (such as before workouts) yet soothe. And soothing can be a great thing in this case! I find by applying 2-3 drops in the palm of my hand and inhaling 6-8 big inhalations, the aroma soothes to settle me down and I find I can wait until the next break or gas station. We can use this same concept for days we are wound up and need that soothing aroma for mood support. (Many think of lavender for this purpose, but I actually prefer peppermint).

Lavender Essential Oil & Lavender Vitality™ Essential Oil

Known as the Swiss Army Knife of oils due to its many uses, Lavender has been used for thousands of years. Its gentle, soothing aroma makes it a favorite and was the "gateway" oil for many of us. Because it's so gentle, it can be used on young to elderly alike with the usual caution of spot testing a small area of skin first. When most people smell a true lavender essential oil, they tend to compare it to the typical lavender on the market used by the food and fragrance industries. These often contain added fragrance and synthetics. Unfortunately, the average person loves the smell (like my daughter did) and bases her decision on the effects of lavender on this cheaper grade of EO containing fragrance versus a pure grade EO like Young Living's lavender essential oil. And that's a shame because the effect a high-grade lavender EO can have for nervous system support is powerful.

Once Karly gave Young Living's lavender a fair try, she told me how amazing the YL oils I had sent her oils were. This came from a non-believer who liked her "perfumey" lavender from the local pharmacy. If YL's lavender could convince a nonbeliever, it must be good! We love lavender in our home for that wonderful mood support along with using it in a multitude of personal care products; it's free of toxins but loaded with fabulous aroma to soothe the body and brain. We diffuse, inhale, and apply lavender topically. Some people like to use lavender internally; they would use Lavender Vitality™ oil for this purpose either in water or a capsule.

If you see the word fragrance on any lavender product, I would avoid it. Fragrance should never need to be in the same bottle as a true lavender oil or in any product in your household. This includes body butters, shampoos, conditioners, Epsom salts, etc. Again, making our own ensures we have zero chemicals. Between lavender, peppermint, and lemon EOs, it would take this entire chapter to list all their uses. This paragraph is a simple explanation of our lavender use; we use it in a multitude of personal care products and diffusing for nervous system support, which is, for us, our most important needs for lavender.

Lemon Essential Oil & Lemon Vitality™ Essential Oil

It's extremely likely all of us have receptor sites loaded with chemicals from our environment, especially any lady who has used synthetic hormones/birth control pills. These chemicals and synthetics are very difficult for the body to break down and eliminate. Since Lemon's cleansing and purifying properties can be great support to our Liver, where we break down estrogens, I would highly recommend you make Lemon Vitality™ Oil as part of your everyday protocol. Based on my readings, the constituents in this oil indicate this should be an absolute for each and every one of us, not only females, to use in capsules or in my water (which I do daily).

When I mention Lemon Vitality ™ Oil in my water, people tell me they already squeeze fresh lemon in their water. There are some big differences here.

- The juice of a lemon is taken from the pulp with an acid PH (pH 2-3) as it is made up of about 5% citric acid. This can bother a person's tummy, especially first thing in the morning.

- Lemon essential oil is derived from the rind and is pH neutral; it does not contain citric acid.

- Because lemon essential oil comes from the rind of the lemon, it possesses different constituents than the juice. Essential oil contains about 70 percent d-limonene, which is something every single human body should welcome.

- It takes seventy-five lemons to produce enough oil for YL's standard sized 15-ml bottle. How much juice would a person have to squeeze from a fresh lemon to equal the power of a few drops of essential oil in their morning water?

Now let's talk about this essential oil's additional benefits.

- It has cleansing and purifying properties.
- It can uplift a person's mood.
- Since it's non-acidic, it can support healthy PH levels.
- Lemon vitality can support healthy digestion. (What is part of the digestive system? Your liver!)

How to Use

For Lemon Vitality™ Oil, drop in water, Ningxia Red, salad dressings, over avocados, etc. The uses are as many as your imagination on this one. Please remember to only use *glass* containers, not plastic when using lemon (or any citrus essential oils) in your water, other drinks, or foods as the lemon can erode the sides of the glass. This means, if you drink from plastic and use Lemon Vitality™ Oil, you are defeating your purpose of reducing chemicals.

For lemon oil, diffuse or inhale for a mood elevator. Add to lotion for support of healthy skin (but remember *not* to use if your skin will be exposed to sun as lemon can irritate or pigment skin). Use in cleaners for a clean smell, bright shine, and dissolve sticky residue. Remember lemon oil can damage surfaces so always spot treat first.

StressAway Oil Blend™

The name kind of says it all on this one. It really is a great blend of the oils of copaiba, vanilla, lime, cedarwood, ocotea, and lavender; it's perfect to help with life's daily challenges. The smell of these oils combined into one blend is gentle and very soothing, which makes it a great one for young children and elderly as all of us in between those ages. Diffuse, inhale, or use the roll-on StressAway™ to apply to brainstem area (top of neck right under the skull) whenever you feel the need.

Release Oil Blend™

This is a very appropriately named blend that can be considered support for positive emotions as well as releasing negative emotions. Why? Release™ is a blend with a relaxing aroma that facilitates the ability to let go of anger and frustration. It also promotes harmony and balance. In traditional Chinese medicine, it is often thought that emotions unresolved will manifest in the most susceptible part of the body. Anger, hurt, and resentment are emotions too many hold in the body. We go along from day to day functioning fairly well. But, at some point, when the organ is weak, the emotions stored will manifest into health issues. According to Chinese medicine, as the liver is supported and cleansed, it will allow for the release of toxins but also emotions. This makes total sense to me and is a big reason I love the

Release Blend. I apply two drops topically over the liver and inhale usually once or twice a day if I have a day where I feel a need to release emotions holding me back.

JuvaFlex™ Oil Blend

Can you imagine never cleaning the filter on your furnace or air conditioning unit? The predicted life of that system would be greatly shortened, wouldn't it? This is how we need to think of our liver; it's a badly overworked, overburdened organ that is a part of the digestive system. The less support it gets, the worse it functions and, honestly, the worse we look. An often-overlooked function of the liver that we discussed in the main body of this book is aiding in our hormone balance. It's function of synthesizing and metabolizing estrogen—including powerful, unwanted estrogens—is a huge part of hormone processing. There simply is no way around the fact if we have poor liver health, we have poor hormone balance, which can contribute to some of the severe female conditions we see today.

In addition, the more toxins that remain in the body, the more fat cells the body need to retain for toxins storage. If we want less fat, we need fewer toxins in the body? Who is in charge of these chemicals and toxins? Our liver, the largest internal organ in the human body, works for us to filter and send toxins/chemicals further down the chain for elimination from the precious vessel it was designed to protect—your body. Thus, the saying "love our liver." It is surely loving on you with its tremendous job of filtering it does. Let's return the favor by supporting it by eating organic and non-GMO food, using chemical-free personal care products, AND giving the liver support to do the rigorous job it has been assigned from the man above. Let's keep in mind our interior health is reflected on the exterior. If we want clear eyes, clear skin, and an overall vibrant look, we are tremendously better to invest in our insides than the pricey creams at the cosmetic counter.

Out of all Young Living's Juva-labeled products, JuvaFlex™ is my choice for daily use for healthy liver support. The key to this oil blend is that it's gentle but gives great support for healthy liver function. Combining the single oils of fennel, geranium, rosemary, Roman chamomile, blue tansy, and helichrysum essential oils, JuvaFlex® is affordable yet supportive to our liver. It is approved for topical use, so I apply 2-3 drops daily over my liver or on the VitalFlex point of the feet and rub in circular motion to help drive it in. Because there are multiple Young Living Juva products, I will discuss them to help with any confusion. I will list the rest of the Juva products and descriptions (including the powerhouse Juva Cleanse™ Blend) after I am done listing the oils and supplements we use in our daily protocol.

MultiGreens™

I wasn't a big user of this supplement until I saw the benefits for Karly as she added this one as part of her plan for maintaining wellness and giving her energy levels and vitality. This caused me to really look at the ingredients in MultiGreens™ and, once again, I had to admire Gary Young's ability to combine ingredients that work in synergy together to create one excellent supplement. What *I love* about MultiGreens™ is it contains pacific kelp, which is a great source of iodine (thyroid support), spirulina (which contains chlorophyll-rich in magnesium,) bee pollen, and amino acids. All this is combined with essential oils of geranium, rosemary, lemon, lemongrass, and melissa oil for one powerhouse of a greens supplement!

Thyromin™

This supplement capsule pairs beautifully with EndoFlex™ and Progessence Plus™ for supporting our endocrine system. Our adrenals and thyroid are often the first glands to feel the effect of estrogen dominance, poor gut health, and stressful lifestyles.

It is, by far, wiser to support a healthy gland with YL products than to try and repair a damaged one. How do we support? Care for our gut to reduce inflammation, and reduce stress and toxins to avoid a burden on the adrenals and thyroid. Once these things bring you above the wellness line, support with EndoFlex, Progessence Plus, and Thyromin™ (This product does contain iodine and is a blend of porcine glandular extracts, herbs, amino acids, minerals, Vitamin E, kelp, CoQ10 and therapeutic-grade essential oils of spearmint, peppermint, myrtle, and myrrh). I use one capsule in the morning and one in the evening on empty stomach.

OmegaGize™

This is Young Living's fish oil. We have discussed the importance of healthy cholesterol for brain support (the brain is our most cholesterol-rich organ of the human body) as well as support for function of our endocrine system. The whole chain of steroid hormones comes from cholesterol, which means high-quality fish oil is vital to proper hormone function and overall wellness support. In addition, studies show it's vital to have fats for optimum Vitamin-D absorption. Thus, the beauty of having both fish oil fats as well as Vitamin D combined in this one capsule. Add in the CoQ10-an essential enzyme for cell energy and you have an excellent "fish oil on steroids". In addition, it contains an essential oil blend of clove, German chamomile, and spearmint to create a supplement that, used daily, supports normal brain, heart, eye, and joint health. You could use another brand of high-quality fish oil, but you would be hard-pressed to ever find the blend of ingredients with the power to help support the body as well as OmegaGize.

Super B™ Vitamin

Super B™ was one I made sure Karly used daily in her wellness support since stress literally sucks the B vitamins right out of us. Stress comes in many forms including physical pain, emotional stress, surgery, life changes—anything that causes us worry or concern. B vitamins are not stored in the body and must be replenished daily either through our food or a high-quality B vitamin. That's why it's important to get a high quality B vitamin that contains all eight essential, energy-boosting B vitamins (B1, B2, B3, B5, B6, B7, B9, and B12) rather than looking for one or two specific ones. Recently reformulated, it now features Orgen-FA®, a natural folate source derived from lemon peels and methylcobalamin, a more bioavailable source of B12. Combined with nutmeg essential oil and bioavailable chelated minerals such as magnesium, manganese, selenium, and zinc, Super B not only assists in maintaining healthy energy levels, it also supports mood and cardiovascular and cognitive function.

Chapter Twenty-Four: Essential Oils for Digestive Support

I am going to end my must-haves with the digestive support products I use daily. Young Living has so many products and oils for digestive support, it can make your head spin. Does that indicate the importance they place on supporting the digestive system? You bet! It's another reason I love this company. Therefore, I will focus on the ones I use as well as a few related ones. Keep in mind, from our main portion of the book, how vital digesting food to avoid inflammation and damage to the gut lining is for support of the digestive system. In addition, remember the importance of probiotics (Young Livings probiotic is called Life ®, which we will discuss) for supporting the immune system. We will start with my daily favorites and then discuss the related products in case they might sound like a good fit for you.

DiGize™ and DiGize Vitality™ Oil Blend

I tell people to think "DI-Gize=DI-GESTION" to hopefully help them remember what this oil's intended use. It's been a mainstay (and favorite) in our home for years. If you haven't tried it, that's a shame and let's hopefully remedy that problem. Why? Because I don't want you to miss out on a wonderful EO blend for you and your family to support overall wellness and healthy digestion. If I were handing out free oils, this is the one I would make sure went to every household. The oils in this blend are comprised of tarragon, ginger, peppermint, juniper, fennel, lemongrass, anise, and patchouli. The soothing combo for supporting not only the tummy but the entire digestive system.

Ancient cultures—and still many cultures today—chew fennel seeds after a meal to aid in support of a healthy digestive system. Every single oil in this blend has constituents that can support healthy digestion. Therefore, even though I use Essentialzyme4™ (discussion coming up next), I still use a few drops of DiGize Vitality™ in a small amount of water just prior to my meals. If you forget, you can always do this after a meal too. I think it pairs well with the digestive enzymes in Essentialzyme4™ perform better. You can also use this in a capsule—one drop of the blend with four drops of carrier oil (olive, coconut, any light, organic oil, or Young Living's V-6 blend of carrier oils) and swallow prior to, with, or after meals. DiGize™ Oil (not the Vitality label) is great to rub topically for little ones (dilute slightly) or even adults who need support after eating something that didn't agree with them.

Essentialzyme4™

This is the digestive enzyme product of Young Living that I use the most. The constituents in Essentialzyme4 ™ are great for people who eat more salads and whole foods and not as much meat. It contains a fabulous blend of essential oils to complement the variety of digestive enzymes. Having EO oils paired with enzymes in the capsules is as good as it gets in my mind. Each serving comes in a foil packet with two capsules; the plant enzymes capsule releases in the stomach while the animal-based enzymes capsule releases in the large intestine. The large intestine is the final section of the gastrointestinal tract that performs the vital task of absorbing water and vitamins while converting digested food into feces. That's a big job. The enzymes in the second capsule help the large intestine with support for the all-important task of absorbing the vitamins from our food. It's super handy to toss one of these foil packets of these enzymes in my purse at all times so that if I eat out, I always have my enzymes with me. This product contains bee pollen to which some people can have an allergic reaction; start out slowly and ease into using.

Essentialzyme™

This is another of Young Living's digestive enzymes. They have multiple types of enzymes, but if you had to choose one for heavier meals or with meat this might be the one. One difference in Essentialzyme™ versus Essentialzyme4™ is that Essentialzyme™ contains HCL (hydrochloric acid) meant to digest heavier meals and meat as well as pancreatic enzymes for pancreas support. It is a good overall digestive enzyme that includes EOs— something you won't likely find in a commercial digestive enzyme at the retail store. The YL description for this product reads, "Essentialzyme is a multienzyme caplet formulated to improve digestive health, enzyme activity, and pancreatic function while reducing pancreatic stress." I list the description mainly because I like that they mention the pancreas. As we discussed earlier, the pancreas secretes our master hormone (insulin) and, due to high sugar and carb diets, this is an organ badly overworked from the food side of things like our liver from the chemicals to which we are exposed. Both organs need all the help we can give them. In this case, we cut sugar and carbs and use Essentialzyme.

How to Use
You can take one tablet with meals to assist with digestion, especially meals high in protein. Take in between meals to improve overall enzyme activity

and support healthy pancreatic function.

Detoxyme™

This digestive enzymes supplement has become my new favorite. For those who need a little help to get their daily "chores" done, this is the one. Although ComforTone is great as well, I find Detoxyme™ to have more effect. However, it is not intended for daily, long-term use as it's fairly powerful and may be used in conjunction with a cleansing or detoxifying program. This is intended for the relief of occasional symptoms such as fullness, pressure, bloating, gas, pain, and/or minor cramping that may occur after eating. Read package instructions and warnings for use.

ComforTone®

This is a great digestive system support capsule of herbs and essential oils that I have definitely included in my protocol when I need a little support getting things moving. I especially find it useful when traveling and the system just isn't moving along as it should. It is gentle (more gentle than Detoxyme™) but effective. The only reason I wouldn't use it on an everyday, long-term basis is because we really should have a digestive system that moves along well on its own through diet and proper gut health. Therefore, this one is great for an occasional cleanup or motivator for our colon but don't depend on it to replace a good diet full of fiber. The description from YL's website states it well, "ComforTon® contains an effective combination of herbs and essential oils that support the health of the digestive system by eliminating residues from the colon and enhancing its natural ability to function optimally. It also promotes liver, gall bladder, and stomach health." For usage, follow the directions on the bottle.

Life 5™ Probiotic

We discussed (repeatedly) how vital proper microbiome balance is to support of our overall body immune system. We can get support through fermented foods and also through probiotic capsules. What's important is to get a variety of strains in your supplement. Life 5™ has five clinically proven probiotic strains including two advanced super strains to enhance intestinal health, sustain energy, and improve immunity. Life 5™ contains ten billion active cultures and improves colonization up to ten times.

It's important for children as well as adults to get microbiome support, especially if we have ever been on antibiotics as the body will need support to retain balance. For young children, open the Life 5™ capsule and pour half on their cereal or in their drink. For nursing babies, mama can open the capsule and apply some of the powder on baby's cheeks and tongues baby gets the good bacteria.

This concludes my discussion of what we use in our daily protocol. As you will note, we use some from the list on each of the systems (nervous, digestive, and endocrine) listed near the beginning of the chapter. Every person will find what products are most helpful to them depending on the area they want to support. Space will just not allow listing and discussing all the oils/products. Before we conclude this chapter, I will list a few more products out of the digestive and endocrine system lists that I have found helpful. This way you will have a slight introduction to a few more possibilities:

Prenolone + ™

This is a cream that has some wonderful skin-moisturizing constituents. It

389

also supports the body in its production of pregnenolone, the precursor to progesterone. I have discussed pregnenolone as an important area of endocrine system support. Keep in mind we are not adding with this product, we are offering support to the systems of the body involved.

CortiStop®

I almost included CortiStop® capsules as one of my products for daily protocol because I really find it to be an excellent product. However, because it's not recommended for long-term daily use, I waited to include it here. Why is it a great product? Because, according to the YL website, "CortiStop Women's is a proprietary dietary supplement designed to help the body balance its cortisol levels to maintain its natural balance and harmony." Supporting healthy levels is a much smarter strategy than trying to re-gain a healthy level. Obviously, no product will take care of whatever is causing elevated cortisol. It is vital you address whatever that issue might be. However, offering occasional support to help maintain the balance is a nice benefit to this supplement. Use according to bottle instructions.

The Juvas

We have already discussed JuvaFlex™ blend earlier in this section since it's one of my daily use oils. However, I did want to provide a little clarification on the other Young Living Juva products since they are designed to support our liver and I surely do love anything we can do to support this underappreciated organ. When you are ready to give the liver more or different support than just JuvaFlex™ Blend, you can consider the following options.

390

Juva Cleanse® Oil Blend

If JuvaFlex™ is the gentle, daily blend, JuvaCleanse™ is the powerhouse. It contains three single oils! Helichrysum essential oil has restorative properties. Remember our liver is the only organ in the human body that regenerates itself, which takes loads of energy. Restorative support is badly needed! Also in this blend is ledum essential oil (think L for liver health), and celery essential oil, which is also known for its support to the liver. We are exposed to more than just daily chemicals at times in our lives like metals such as mercury in silver amalgam fillings, metal carriers in medical injections, toxins in the air. The liver has a big job to do, and sometimes it needs extra support to do its job. This is where Juva Cleanse comes in. I personally wouldn't use it until you've done some other support work to lay the foundation for liver support (such as JuvaFlex™). But once you are ready to work on a cleanse for your liver, JuvaCleanse® is a great product. Use in a capsule one drop oil to four parts carrier or in a glass with four ounces of liquid such as goat or rice milk.

JuvaPower® Powder

This is a powder form of delivery for our liver support with digestive cleansing. Rich in liver-supporting nutrients, JuvaPower® is an antioxidant vegetable powder complex and is one of the richest sources of acid-binding foods with intestine-cleansing benefits.

JuvaSpice®

Just like its name implies, JuvaSpice™ is a powder for seasoning food. It contains great liver support ingredients.

JuvaTone®

JuvaTone® comes in a tablet form and is an excellent source of choline, which makes it a good choice for those on high-protein diets. JuvaTone® also contains inositol and di-methionine, which help with the body's normal excretion functions—a vital function in our toxin-ridden diet and environment.

When all is said and done, the key is to make yourself aware of the importance of liver support as well as the variety of products available to deliver that support. My advice is to start out gently—thus, my choice of JuvaFlex™. Use it for a while and then venture off to try some of the other great Juva—liver support—products when you are ready.

A Few Final Favorites

Coriander Essential Oil

This is one of my favorites just because I like how I feel when I use it. It offers support for the digestive system and has also been studied for support it might offer to a healthy pancreas. We have talked extensively on excess sugar that wreaks havoc on our insulin hormone. Insulin is secreted by the pancreas so when it is in a constant state of secreting the insulin hormone, it places high demands on our pancreas. Many body conditions can come about as a result of less than optimum pancreas health. As we change our diets to reduce sugar/grains and bring our pancreas to optimum health, it is then good to support it with coriander. One note on coriander is that I would not use more than 1-2 drops; it is powerful and I respect its power by never using more than the 1-2 drops at one time.

Ylang Ylang

This oil is in most of Young Living's blends for nervous system support and emotional support for good reason. It's a fabulous oil that balances male/female energies and aligns body energy. It's one of my favorites for helping bring my body frequency down a tad on the days I want that support. I use it on my wrists as a non-toxic perfume but no more than one drop as the scent can be overwhelming. Inhale this, diffuse it, and use to nourish positive emotions and reach a state of harmony.

Idaho Balsam Fir

Like almost all the pine oils, Idaho balsam fir has that wonderful aroma that has a calming, grounding effect. It's great for those of us who need to bring things down a notch when our thoughts are racing.

Idaho Blue Spruce

This is a favorite oil for many "manly" men with Young Living; the scent and effect for feeling manly is powerful. Our 89-year-old friend George loves this oil. If the scent of this one can keep him feeling manly at his age, that's a good oil! Once again, as a pine oil, it has the soothing aroma of helping us feel grounded and strengthened.

Shutran™

This is another favorite often worn as a cologne for many men. The scent and effect for feeling manly is powerful. Once again, this is a favorite of our friend George, who applies it daily to his wrists and neck.

Prostate Health®

The thought process of "far better to support than try to fix" is especially important for men and their prostate. In my mind, all men should have the support of Prostate Health. Over half of all men will develop a prostate disorder in their lifetime. Prostate Health supports a healthy male glandular system (with the prostate one very important gland) and helps maintain normal, healthy, prostate function. Saw Palmetto's powerful fatty acids combined with essential oils and natural pumpkin seed oil supports a healthy inflammation response.

Bergamot

Bergamot has a light citrusy scent, which can be both uplifting and relaxing when diffused. The same principle applies here as for balsam fir. Soothe the brain and emotions to ease the burden on other body systems. Bergamot is highly photosensitive; do not apply to areas that will have sun exposure. I like to say "put it where the sun don't shine."

Cedarwood

This contains the highest level of sesquiterpenes of all the EOs. This is a great oil for supporting the nervous system and enhancing focus. This is a good one for children (and adults) who can't seem to stay on task. Its aroma creates a calming yet powerful environment. Apply to the brainstem area and/or the VitalFlex point of the brain, which is the bottom of each big toe.

Black Pepper Vitality

We discussed the benefits of black pepper spice and why it's been highly valued since ancient times for flavoring as well as nutrient absorption. It's why pepper is always on a table along with salt. I like to add a drop of Black Pepper Vitality to my green drinks, lettuce salads, even my kefir and berries mixture. The taste of it is very mild and, since I want the benefits, it's in my foods.

My "Trifecta of Oils" (Frankincense, Neroli, and Galbanum)

This is a blend I absolutely love and use daily. I apply to the crown of my head for opening the Crown Chakra energy effect as well as the physical aspect. Did you know the head has a glymphatic system for elimination for our nervous system? According to the 2015 research "The Glymphatic System: A Beginner's Guide" from the School of Medicine and Dentistry at the University of Rochester,

> The glymphatic system is a recently discovered macroscopic waste clearance system that utilizes a unique system of perivascular tunnels, formed by astroglial cells, to promote efficient elimination of soluble proteins and metabolites from the central nervous system.

Support of the central nervous system is an important part of my day. For my last listing of favorite oils, I like to mention this blend I use every morning for setting the tone of the day, balancing energies for maintaining focus throughout the day *and* as support of a healthy glymphatic system.

Frankincense is stimulating and elevating to the mind-high in sesquiterpenes, which can help stimulate to help support normal health of the limbic system of the brain (our emotional control center) as well as maintain a normal, healthy hypothalamus, the master gland of the body and one that releases many hormones. Frankincense is widely used to help open the crown chakra for grounding, centering and spiritual connection. The three wise men did not need to give Mary and Joseph instructions on using this powerful oil when they delivered it. In ancient times, it was used for every part of the body for supporting and grounding—from head to toe.

Galbanum is one of the lowest frequency oils but when combined with frankincense its frequency rises dramatically. Its fragrance gives beautiful harmony and balance to the mind. Personally, I find galbanum one of the most grounding of all oils I have used.

Neroli's aroma helps bring everything to focus at that moment. Its influence helps to stabilize our mind, body, and spirit to be in the present moment—neither being concerned about the past nor worrying about the future. Neroli reminds me somewhat of Ylang Ylang for its powerful, sweet aroma and equally powerful effect on the senses.

While the oils in this trio aren't the lower priced oils, I feel they are worth the effect. Start by standing in front of a mirror so you can see how many drops go on your head when applying this blend of oils. Drop each oil on the crown of the head. It's a tad difficult at first when trying to work around hair but just use your fingers to make a part at the back of the head at the crown. After making and holding this part with your fingers, use your other hand to drop your oils onto the part while watching in the mirror to see how many drops come out. I use two drops of each oil. Use frankincense first for opening the crown chakra. After applying your two drops, slide your fingers under the hair so you can put pressure on the scalp; make short, little motions to rub back and forth for a bit to work the oil in. Next do the same with neroli and then galbanum. The order on these two isn't as important, but it is important to use frankincense first. After applying two drops of each oil and rubbing, let it absorb for a minute or two and then end with a tad bit of carrier oil. Apply to your fingers and rub in over the area. I do this to "hold in" the oils. Since oils are molecularly miniscule, this means they evaporate quickly, which is why I like to end with the carrier oil. As all good oilers know, inhale the oils remnants on your fingertips or rub on directly under your nose. If you give this blend a try, I'd love to hear if you like it. Send me an email to the one listed at the end of the book if you wish.

This concludes our discussion of just some of many of Young Living's supplements and essential oils. As I have mentioned, there are a multitude of books and guides on the use of EOs. I encourage you to read all you can, not only on essential oils and the support they can offer the body systems but on your overall health. My hope for you and your family is that you avoid the path we took by removing toxins before they emerge as health issues. Supporting is a far better approach than fixing. Using your EOs to create your own chemical-free products or choosing from Young Living's extensive line of personal care products is an excellent way to avoid the chemicals that must be removed from the environment in which we and, our family, lives. Choosing to inhale a soothing scent over popping a pill to relieve life's daily pressures is an excellent habit to develop for both you and your children. Supporting health with EOs rather than trying to regain health is a much wiser way to work with our body. Finally, choosing to be the specialist in your health and your family's health is a life decision you will never regret. Essential oils are an excellent way to support and take charge of your health. Enjoy learning all you can. They are amazing, fascinating, and fun. Enjoy!

Reference Sites to Obtain More Information on Essential Oils

Abundant Health: www.abundanthealth4u.com

Life Science Publishers: www.discoverlsp.com

Crown Diamond Tools: www.http://crowndiamondtools.soundconcepts.com

Easy Recipes using Essential Oils

(All recipes use organic food and liquids.)

Popcorn with EO butter topping

When I do indulge in popcorn, I use:

o Air Popper popcorn popper—(If you use a stovetop pan or Stir Crazy Popper and organic, refined coconut oil)

o Organic popcorn

o Melted, blended combo of butter (organic, from grass-fed cows) and organic coconut oil

o Vitality™ Essential Oil favorite flavor *after* removing from heat—some suggestions are Cinnamon, Black Pepper, Dill

o Sea salt

o Essentialzyme-4 digestive enzymes (Popcorn is a tough one for the digestive system to break down!)

Black Pepper and Cinnamon in Hemp Protein Drink

o Organic, Hi-Fiber Hemp Protein (I like Nutiva® brand)

o Water, Coconut or Almond milk (Make sure your milk has no carrageenan in it.)

o One drop each of Black Pepper Vitality™ Oil (aids absorption of nutrients) and Cinnamon Vitality™ Oil (Great help with the flavor to help the Hemp go down!)

Mix all in a shaker bottle and drink. Shake often. Plant protein is by far easier on the kidneys. Hemp fibers bind to toxins and metals (super important) in the body to help carry them from the body. This is a super easy way to get something into the body in a hurry when you are on the run. I won't brag about taste but surely good for us.

All content regarding Essential Oils was written by Teri A. Ringham, Member # 1089748, a Young Living Independent Distributor. Content was not sponsored nor approved by Young Living. Please view and abide my disclaimer at the beginning of this book and chapter on Essential Oils.

TO CONTACT TERI:

Email: info@teriswellnesstips.com
Facebook: Teris Wellness Tips
Website: TerisWellnessTips.com

FOR ESSENTIAL OILS USERS:

Email: teri@younglivingoils.com
Facebook: Younger Living Oils
Website: youngerlivingoils.com
Young Living Member #1089748

Acknowledgments

Who ever knew writing a book was such an undertaking? Not me! What an eye-opening experience this has been. I could never have imagined the time involved in creating a book. That being said, this process has involved many emotions. I've felt sadness as my research for this book reinforces to me the escalating number of health issues in not only our elderly but in our younger generation as well. It's also caused frustration as this writing and research emphasizes the dollars invested by powerful companies with little regard for human lives and especially our children's lives. I've felt grateful for the opportunity to reach out and possibly open readers' minds to the chemicals in their diets and personal environments in hopes they make a stand to remove them. And finally, I'm incredibly thankful for the people who have enabled me to branch out into the unknown territory of putting my thoughts, acquired knowledge, and beliefs in this book.

Marty Ringham, my lifelong partner and husband, who has weathered the good as well as the bad in this life right along with me. Your "get it done" attitude and confidence in my work motivated me to attempt this book even when I wanted to make excuses. Thank you for your unwavering love and support of this project that is near and dear to my heart. Without you, it would never have been possible.

George Dutra, my adopted father, spiritual guide, and best friend. How could I dare disappoint? Your encouragement and avid faith in my abilities buoyed me when I most needed it and allowed no room for anything other than success. Your heart, energy, and vitality at eighty-nine years old coupled with your fifty-six years of zero doctor appointments are testimony that the results of caring for ourselves naturally does justify the means! You are a shining example that being older but living younger is a very real possibility.

Adam Ringham, an intelligent young man, wonderful father to little Tolly, and my son who set the bar high by writing his own successful book. Your confidence of putting your knowledge on paper was a guide and motivator during the times my energy waned. Our shared love for natural health and impassioned frustration at the inequities of the system make me proud to be your mother (and also make for some interesting dinner conversations).

Tony Ringham, my son who follows his own drummer. We haven't quite brought you into the fold on total natural health, but you know we will keep trying. Your quick wit, intelligence, and commitment to grow a successful business make me proud to be your mother. You have been an inspiration to me on what we can accomplish when we apply ourselves. (P.S. We won't tell Pixie I might recommend bacon for its healthy cholesterol!)

Karly Ringham, your inner light continued to shine in spite of the wrongs in your world. You are my inspiration not only for this book but also for those who struggle. There *can* be hope at the end of every tunnel. Your ability to put one foot in front of the other during your darkest times spurred me to continue searching for answers even when it appeared there were none. No pain is greater than a mother watching her child struggle. No joy is greater than a mother seeing her child happy. This mother is eternally thankful to be in a place of joy at this time. Shine on, my daughter!

Finally, to my readers. Many of you have encouraged and pushed me to write this book. Your belief and confidence that it may be helpful to you inspires and honors me. My prayers go out to each and every one of you that you will find some source of motivation within this written material to create the necessary determination needed for a positive change in your life.

About the Author

Teri Ringham's varied background has led her full circle in her passion for fitness and health. Avidly involved in varsity and state sports competitions throughout her school years, she was an NCAA national qualifier for women's track and field pentathlon held at UCLA in her freshman and sophomore years of college. Her B.A. in Business Administration was obtained from Upper Iowa University and she holds a real estate broker's license in both FL and MN. When her daughter was diagnosed with an autoimmune condition, Teri's passion for business and real estate waned as she engulfed herself in health research and accessing health professionals in her quest for a cure.

Currently immersed in a holistic lifestyle, Teri holds a Reiki Level One certification, certification from the Institute of Nutritional Health Leadership, is a speaker at wellness conferences, and schedules consultations for Gut & Hormone Wellness at her office at the BeWell Center in Naples FL. She is a self-professed natural health fanatic who shuttles between her Florida and Minnesota homes with her yappy dog Sailor in tow. Teri is the proud parent of three children and married 39 years to her extremely supportive husband, Marty.

TO CONTACT TERI:

Email: info@teriswellnesstips.com
Facebook: Teris Wellness Tips
Website: TerisWellnessTips.com